Well-Being Therapy

Giovanni A. Fava

Well-Being Therapy

Treatment Manual and Clinical Applications

6 figures, and 66 tables, 2016

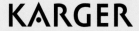

Basel · Freiburg · Paris · London · New York · Chennai · New Delhi · Bangkok · Beijing · Shanghai · Tokyo · Kuala Lumpur · Singapore · Sydney

Prof. Giovanni A. Fava
Professor of Clinical Psychology
University of Bologna, Italy
Clinical Professor of Psychiatry
State University of New York at Buffalo, USA

Università di Bologna
Dipartimento di Psicologia
viale Berti Pichat 5
IT–40127 Bologna (Italy)
E-Mail giovanniandrea.fava@unibo.it

Library of Congress Cataloging-in-Publication Data

Names: Fava, Giovanni A. (Giovanni Andrea), author.
Title: Well-being therapy : treatment manual and clinical applications /
   Giovanni A. Fava.
Description: Basel ; New York : Karger, 2016. | Includes bibliographical
   references and index.
Identifiers: LCCN 2015047374| ISBN 9783318058215 (soft cover : alk. paper) |
   ISBN 9783318058222 (electronic version)
Subjects: | MESH: Mental Disorders--therapy | Mental Health |
   Psychotherapy--methods
Classification: LCC RC480.5 | NLM WM 400 | DDC 616.89/14--dc23 LC record available at
http://lccn.loc.gov/2015047374

© Copyright 2016 by Giovanni A. Fava. Published by S. Karger AG, Basel
www.karger.com
Printed in Germany on acid-free and non-aging paper (ISO 9706) by Kraft Druck, Ettlingen
ISBN 978–3–318–05821–5
e-ISBN 978–3–318–05822–2

Contents

Part III: APPLICATIONS

The information in this volume is not intended as a substitute for consultation with physicians. Each individual's health concern should be evaluated by a qualified professional.

For further information see also: www.well-being-therapy.com

Foreword

The publication of this first book on Well-Being Therapy (WBT) is a landmark event. Giovanni Fava's pioneering work in developing this powerful and richly layered psychotherapy has stimulated a series of research studies that have shown robust effectiveness for psychiatric disorders. But until now clinicians have not had a manual that spells out the details of treatment delivery and gives specific, session-by-session instructions on how to put WBT into action. The book should promote wider use of a therapy that offers great promise for resolving symptoms and achieving personal balance.

My introduction to WBT came at an international conference where I had the good fortune to attend a workshop given by Dr. Fava. All I knew in advance of the workshop was that WBT had shown strong results in studies of residual depression and relapse prevention, and that it focuses more on developing positive thoughts and emotions than traditional cognitive behavior therapy (CBT). I was soon to discover that WBT goes far beyond positive psychology and offers a unique treatment method grounded in a multidimensional model of human potential.

Among the revelations in that first workshop with Dr. Fava, I learned that a practical strategy of keeping a log of well-being experiences could improve mood and reduce symptoms of depression. Having practiced CBT for many years prior to my exposure to WBT, I typically encouraged patients to do thought records that focused on identifying negative or troubling cognitions and emotions. Had I been training them to sharpen their skills in looking for the negative? If they were already accomplished at locking into distressing, self-condemning thoughts, did they need a 180° turn in their thinking? I wasn't ready to abandon the core tenants of CBT. They had helped many of my patients overcome depression and anxiety. And there is an abundance of empirical evidence for the effectiveness of CBT. However, the workshop primed me to try adding WBT methods to standard CBT techniques.

My first attempt to enrich treatment with WBT concepts was encouraging. I chose a difficult-to-treat situation – a young woman who had been stuck in bipolar depression for over 2 years despite intensive pharmacotherapy. She was living with her parents and unable to work. With crippling low self-esteem, a sense of stagnation and hopelessness for the future, and severely restricted social relationships, she had deep problems in most of the areas of functioning targeted in WBT. Her initial foray with a well-being log was tentative but productive.

She had been invited to attend a wedding of a friend from high school, but was hesitant to accept the invitation. Yet, she decided to try to shop for a dress to wear to the wedding. Her initial entry on a well-being log captured some experiences that otherwise might have hardly registered in her consciousness. She wrote that the clerk, an older woman, had paid special attention to her and was very kind and supportive in helping her find a suitable outfit for the event. The clerk's encouraging voice and warm smile gave her a sense of well-being that she wouldn't have fully appreciated without taking the time to log it.

As the therapy progressed, we built upon this first experience to help her recognize and sustain many other episodes of well-being. Eventually such experiences became embedded naturally in her days without the need for logging. In addition to using standard CBT exposure strategies for overcoming patterns of avoidance, we worked on building her self-confidence and self-efficacy with the well-being method that Dr. Fava describes for improving autonomy, personal growth, and other key domains of functioning. The outcome was excellent. At the time of writing this Foreword, she has been free of depressive symptoms for over 7 years, has been working successfully at a demanding job, is living independently, and is engaged to be married. Although all of my attempts at using WBT have not met with this high degree of success, most patients have benefitted. And I have incorporated WBT concepts into my routine work with patients.

The focus of WBT on six domains of personal functioning gives it an appealing depth that may not be realized in traditional CBT. As Dr. Fava notes, these domains (environmental mastery, personal growth, purpose in life, autonomy, self-acceptance, and positive relations with others) were detailed (in close to the current form used in WBT) by Jahoda in *Current Concepts of Positive Mental Health* published in 1958. However, there were no attempts to operationalize these constructs into a therapeutic approach until Dr. Fava treated his first case in 1994 and began research that would culminate in his first publication on WBT in 1998.

Although standard CBT may include methods that target some of the domains (e.g., environmental mastery, autonomy, and self-acceptance), attention to domains such as personal growth, purpose in life, and positive relations with others sets WBT apart as a treatment with a broad, growth-oriented treatment philosophy. This comprehensive perspective on human functioning could link WBT to other valuable methods such as logotherapy, an existentially based method developed by Victor Frankl, and interpersonal psychotherapy. In this first treatment manual on WBT, Dr. Fava gives the greatest detail on the early and middle phases of treatment when well-being diaries and related strategies are used to identify and sustain positive experiences. This alignment toward the more pragmatic and readily conceptualized elements of WBT is understandable and welcome in an initial manual. I look forward to future books that explore the nuances of WBT in later phases that help patients achieve potential and balance in all six domains of functioning.

Another appealing feature of WBT is its easy integration with other treatment approaches. As Dr. Fava explains in the book, WBT is typically performed as part of a package with traditional CBT methods such as cognitive restructuring, behavioral activation, and exposure and response prevention. Pharmacotherapy also can be a useful component of the overall treatment plan with WBT. In *Breaking Free from Depression: Pathways to Wellness* – a self-help guide I wrote with my daughter, Laura McCray, MD – WBT methods are presented (along with standard CBT, medication, and other evidence-based approaches) as one of the key strategies that can be used in an individualized plan to overcome depression.

Research to date on WBT has centered on depression, generalized anxiety disorder, and cyclothymia. But the core features of the approach suggest that treatment methods could be extended to a variety of other indications such as bipolar disorder, psychoses, and helping patients with symptoms of medical illnesses. Modifications in length and/or focus of treatment might be required. To give one example, treatment of bipolar depression might be performed by a psychiatrist who adds WBT methods to pharmacotherapy over many brief sessions to address chronic symptoms of the mood disorder. I used this modification of WBT in twice-monthly to monthly sessions for more than a year with the patient I described earlier.

In treatment of the chronic phase of schizophrenia, some studies have shown that CBT methods are helpful for both the positive and negative symptoms of the disorder. Could a well-being approach assist patients with psychoses who have been stabilized on medication and have residual symptoms? In a long-term clinic I established for patients taking clozapine, we typically spend part of the treatment sessions identifying activities that stimulate a sense of well-being, and we discuss themes of personal meaning, positive interpersonal relationships, and other domains identified in WBT. Relapse and rehospitalization rates have been very low in this group of patients, and many have developed an adaptive perspective that helps them understand and cope with their chronic condition.

An example of a potential treatment application of WBT in the area of medical illness and/or psychosomatic medicine is chronic pain. Could well-being logs from the initial phase of therapy help a person with chronic pain recognize, savor, and prolong experiences that counterbalance and reduce suffering from the medical condition? Could the later phases of WBT help this person tap strengths to build autonomy, self-confidence, and a sense of purpose in the face of the illness? If such changes could be achieved, would the person have a greater level of authentic well-being – not only reduction of pain, or an increased ability to experience happiness, but an overarching, metapsychological well-being that enriches his or her life and limits the impact and reach of pain?

An additional idea for the expansion of WBT is to embrace technological advances in treatment delivery. Work on development and testing of computer-assisted CBT has expanded rapidly in recent years and has shown excellent results in many studies. The goals of computer-assisted CBT include improving access to effective treatment, reducing cost of therapy, enhancing the therapy experience with multimedia learning experiences, and providing tools for tracking and promoting progress. Programs have been developed for depression, anxiety disorders, eating disorders, substance abuse, chronic pain, and other conditions. WBT methods could potentially be provided via fully developed computer programs for treatment or mobile apps that could augment the efforts of human therapists and help clinicians treat more patients with available time.

With the publication of this treatment manual, a new phase in the development of WBT begins. Guidelines are now laid out for clinicians to use this inventive approach in everyday practice. Dissemination among much larger populations of patients can be envisioned. Development of well-being methods for more diverse clinical problems can be projected and supported with a core text on basic theories and procedures. Research on treatment outcome in depression, anxiety, and a variety of other conditions can be anticipated. And innovative delivery methods with computer technology can be conceptualized. Patients and therapists owe a debt of gratitude to Giovanni Fava for introducing WBT into the family of effective psychiatric treatments.

Jesse H. Wright, MD, PhD, Louisville, Ky.

Preface

This book is both the first full account and a manual for a specific psychotherapeutic strategy for increasing psychological well-being: Well-Being Therapy (WBT).

The first part describes how it developed and how it was implemented. The second part outlines the type of assessment that is necessary for its application and provides a session-by-session treatment manual. Finally, the third part deals with the current indications of WBT based on controlled studies and other potential applications, with descriptions of clinical cases.

For this book, I am indebted in particular to Jenny Guidi, PhD; Elena Tomba, PhD; Emanuela Offidani, PhD; Jesse H. Wright, MD; Seung K. Park, MD; Fiammetta Cosci, MD, PhD; Chiara Rafanelli, MD, PhD; and Nicoletta Sonino, MD (my wife), who provided important feedback and encouragement.

Giovanni A. Fava, MD, Bologna/Buffalo, N.Y.

Chapter 1

The Background

When I decided to study medicine, I was not particularly convinced of my choice. The early years were tough: I did not like the topics I was studying in my medical school in Padova, Italy. I was aware that I should consider myself lucky, with a future full of promise, but I kept on wondering whether it was the right choice – until something happened. In those days (early 1970s), medical students had yearly chest X-rays. At the beginning of my third year (medical courses extend over 6 years in Italy), I had mine. A few days later I received a letter stating that there was something wrong and to come back for further checking in a couple of days. My first thought was 'I have tuberculosis'. When I got the letter, I was reading Thomas Mann's *Magic Mountain* and I concluded that this could not be a coincidence: 'I have not been feeling well, recently – I thought – I am more tired than I used to be.' I imagined myself in a sanatorium, far away from my family, friends, and classes. When I eventually went to the clinic for the new check-up, I was a wreck. But at the clinic they told me there must have been a mistake and that my chest was fine. In a matter of seconds, I felt fine and when I left the clinic the sky was blue and there could not be any other medical student happier than I was. I understood that regaining health is a wonderful experience; however, I was never actually sick from a medical viewpoint.

I thus became interested in psychosomatic medicine, a comprehensive framework for assessing the role of psychosocial factors in the development, course, and outcome of illness [1]. However, no one seemed to be interested in psychosomatic medicine in Padova or at other Italian universities. By some lucky circumstance, in 1975 I was able to spend the summer in Rochester, New York, studying with one of the most prominent scholars in the psychosomatic field, George Engel.

The Rochester Experience

George Engel was Professor of Medicine and Professor of Psychiatry at the University of Rochester School of Medicine and Dentistry. Trained as an internist, he had criticized the traditional concept of disease being restricted to what can be understood or recognized by a physician [2]. In other words, only the physician could decide if something is a disease and if a patient can be sick. Engel elaborated a unified concept of health and disease [2]: there is no health and no disease, only a dynamic balance between health and disease. Such a view, expressed in 1960, was subsequently elaborated in the biopsychosocial model [3]. Psychosocial factors are a class of etiological factors in every type of disease, but their relative weight may change from one disease to another, from one patient to another, and even from one episode to another of the same illness in the same patient [4]. It is not that certain diseases, defined as 'functional', lack an explanation, but rather it is our assessment that is inadequate in most clinical encounters [5].

I spent the summer in his medical-psychiatric unit and the experience was for me an endless source of knowledge and inspiration. One day a psychosomatic consultation was requested from a medical ward. With another medical student, Sam, I went to see the patient. She was a lady in her fifties and manifested what appeared to be an unbearable abdominal pain. Medical work-up could not establish a potential cause. Her condition seemed to be deteriorating and explorative surgery was planned in a couple of days (in 1975, today's minimally invasive explorative procedures were not available). Our job was to interview her and get some preliminary history. Dr. Engel would have come later in the day. We started with some questions, but she appeared to be in great pain. Sam and I agreed that it was probably not the right time and should come back with Dr. Engel, which we did. Dr. Engel immediately got her attention and collaboration. At a certain point during the medical interview, he became interested in a scar the patient had. The lady suddenly brightened up and described a past surgical operation. Dr. Engel asked whether she had undergone other surgical interventions. The lady showed other scars and provided detailed descriptions of each surgery. She seemed to forget about her pain. Sam and I could not understand what was going on. She looked so well, while only hours earlier she was in so much pain. Dr. Engel asked how things were going in her life and she replied that after a very troubled time with a lot of problems in her family, things were going reasonably well. When we got out of her room, Dr. Engel told us that the lady had a pain-prone personality and was a surgery addict [6]. When life is treating these patients worst, when circumstances are the hardest, their physical health is likely to be at its best and the individuals are free of pain. When things improve, when some success is imminent, then painful symptoms develop [6]. Sam asked what could be done for these patients. Dr. Engel replied 'Not much, unfortunately. I will speak with her physician and at least this time we will avoid surgery.' Sam and I, with our juvenile wish to help, were very dissatisfied by that answer. I thought 'Maybe one day someone will find the way.'

When the summer was over, I went back to Padova and intended to become like George Engel and be knowledgeable of both internal medicine and psychiatry. In due course, however, I realized that one specialty was already more than I could handle and thus chose psychiatry, the field where most of the psychosomatic researchers came from.

Treating Depression

I started my residency training program in psychiatry in Padova, but my idea was to go back to Rochester to complete my training. Due to certain circumstances that in those days I judged to be unfavorable, I ended up instead in Albuquerque, New Mexico. My teacher and mentor was someone I had met at a psychosomatic conference, Robert Kellner. He had become a psychiatrist after several years as a primary care physician and thus shared something in common with George Engel. He really showed me how the psychosomatic approach could balance pharmacological and psychological therapies in psychiatric practice. Depression was the psychiatric disorder that attracted my attention the most. After 1 year in the southwestern US, I moved to Buffalo, New York, where I was asked to establish a depression unit. I was convinced that depression was essentially an episodic disorder, that there were powerful remedies against it (antidepressant drugs), and chronicity was essentially a consequence of inadequate diagnosis and treatment. Today when I look back on of my views then, I am surprised of my naiveté and clinical blindness. We have become aware that depression is essentially a chronic disorder with multiple acute episodes along its course [7]; however, back then my view was shared by almost every expert in the field.

Working in the US, I had essentially a cross-sectional view of the disorder (I was seeing and treating patients only in the hospital, with little follow-up). However, when I decided to go back to Italy and establish an outpatient clinic at the University of Bologna with opportunities for follow-up, I began to observe that patients I had personally treated with antidepressant drugs and whom I judged to have completely remitted relapsed into depression after some time. What was I missing?

The Concept of Recovery

I became more and more skeptical of the long-term effectiveness of antidepressant drugs to the point that in 1994 I introduced in the literature the hypothesis that these medications could be a cause for chronicity [8]. I was inspired by the 'antibiotic paradox': the best agents for treating bacterial infections are also the best agents for selecting and propagating resistant strains, which persist in the environment even when exposure to the drug is stopped [9]. On the basis of some data that were available, I postulated that long-term use of antidepressant drugs may worsen the long-term outcome and symptomatic expression of illness, decreasing both the likelihood of subsequent response to pharmacological treatment and duration of symptom-free periods [8]. Two decades later the evidence supporting this hypothesis is quite impressive [10], but in those days swimming against the tide of pharmaceutical propaganda was not easy. In Albuquerque, under the guidance of Robert Kellner, I had learned to practice cognitive behavior therapy (CBT). I used it with my depressed patients, whether associated with antidepressant drugs or not, but it did not seem to affect their long-term outcome, as also reported in the literature [7]. This was in striking contrast to the use of CBT in anxiety disorders, where positive and lasting effects could be observed [8].

Meanwhile, more and more studies were pointing to the fact that pharmacological treatment of depression was not solving all the problems and, despite substantial improvement, important residual symptoms were present [11]. Such symptoms included anxiety and irritability in particular, and were associated with impaired functional capacity. Most residual symptoms also occurred in the prodromal phase of illness and might progress to become prodromal symptoms of relapse [11]. As a result, the concept of recovery could not be limited to the abatement of certain symptoms [12]. As Engel indicated [2, 3], health is not simply the absence of disease, but also requires the presence of wellness. We knew how to bring people out of the negative functioning, but regaining psychological well-being was quite different and we did not have a clue about how to achieve it.

Psychological Well-Being

In the mid-1990s, I attended an international conference on psychiatry in Copenhagen, organized by my friend Per Bech, one of the most important and original researchers in psychological assessment of mood disorders [13]. When I met him, he recommended attending a session on quality of life. He explained that one of the speakers was an American developmental psychologist who had some interesting ideas. I went and, as on other occasions, he was right. The speaker was Carol Ryff, who gave an account of her model of psychological well-being, which was a synthesis of various contributions from the literature [14]. She remarked that well-being cannot be equated with happiness or life satisfaction. She had developed a questionnaire for measuring the various dimensions of psychological well-being, the Psychological Well-Being Scales (PWB), which she had applied to nonclinical populations in longitudinal studies [14]. She gave a brief description of each of its six dimensions.

I belong to the endangered species of clinician-researchers who do clinical research as well as assess and treat individual patients. When I examine research constructs, my starting point is always whether these constructs make sense with the patients I see. And Ryff's formulations were able to do this: autonomy (a sense of self-determination), environmental mastery (the capacity to manage effectively one's life), positive interpersonal relationships, personal growth (a sense of continued growth and development), purpose in life (the belief that life is purposeful and meaningful), and self-acceptance (a positive attitude toward self). After her presentation, I started thinking of many patients I had encountered who seemed to have these dimensions impaired or exaggerated with resulting clashes against everyday life. I was surprised that a developmental psychologist could have articulated such deeply clinical formulations.

Many years later I discovered that those dimensions had indeed a clinical root and were developed by Marie Jahoda, Professor of Social Psychology at New York University, in a fantastic book on positive mental health that was published in 1958 [15]. The book was waiting for me in an American library and became a further source of reflection and inspiration. Marie Jahoda had outlined six criteria for positive mental health. In 5 cases these criteria were only slightly different compared to those later outlined by Carol Ryff: autonomy (regulation of behavior from within), environmental mastery, satisfactory interactions with other people and the milieu, the individual's style and degree of growth, development and self-actualization (this was split by Ryff into the dimensions of personal growth and purpose in life), and the attitudes of an individual toward his/her own self (self-perception/acceptance). There was, however, a sixth important dimension whose formulation became particularly important to me at some later point in time: the individual's balance and integration of psychic forces, which encompass both outlook on life and resistance to stress.

Implementing a psychological work aimed at improving psychological well-being appeared to be quite difficult and I did not know how it could be achieved. In 1954, Parloff et al. [16] suggested that the goals of psychotherapy were not necessarily the reduction of symptoms, but instead increased personal comfort and effectiveness. However, there had been a very limited response to these needs in subsequent years. Notable exceptions were Ellis and Becker's *A Guide to Personal Happiness* [17], a modification of rationale-emotive therapy for removing the main blocks to personal happiness (shyness, feeling of inadequacy, feeling of guilt, etc.), Fordyce's program to increase happiness [18], Padesky's work on schema change processes [19], Frisch's quality of life therapy [20], and Horowitz and Kaltreider's work on positive states of mind [21]. Unfortunately, these approaches had not undergone sufficient clinical validation and did not seem to target what I had in mind in terms of psychological well-being.

References

1 Fava GA, Sonino N: Psychosomatic medicine. Int J Clin Practice 2010;64:999–1001.
2 Engel GL: A unified concept of health and disease. Perspect Biol Med 1960;3:459–485.
3 Engel GL: The need for a new medical model. Science 1977;196:129–136.
4 Lipowski ZJ: Physical illness and psychopathology. Int J Psychiatry Med 1974;5:483–497.
5 Fava GA, Sonino N, Wise TN (ed): The Psychosomatic Assessment. Basel, Karger, 2012.
6 Engel GL: 'Psychogenic' pain and the pain-prone patient. Am J Med 1959;26:899–918.
7 Fava GA, Tomba E, Grandi S: The road to recovery from depression. Psychother Psychosom 2007;76:260–265.
8 Fava GA: Do antidepressant and antianxiety drugs increase chronicity in affective disorders? Psychother Psychosom 1994;61:125–131.
9 Levy SB: The Antibiotic Paradox: How Miracle Drugs Are Destroying the Miracle. New York, Plenum, 1992.
10 Andrews PW, Kornstein SG, Halberstadt LJ, Gardner CO, Neale MC: Blue again: perturbational effects of antidepressants suggest monoaminergic homeostasis in major depression. Front Psychol 2011;2:159.
11 Fava GA, Kellner R: Prodromal symptoms in affective disorders. Am J Psychiatry 1991;148:823–830.
12 Fava GA: The concept of recovery in affective disorders. Psychother Psychosom 1996;65:2–13.
13 Bech P: Clinical Psychometrics. Chichester, Wiley, 2012.
14 Ryff CD: Happiness is everything, or is it? Explorations on the meaning of psychological well-being. J Pers Soc Psychol 1989;6:1069–1081.
15 Jahoda M: Current Concepts of Positive Mental Health. New York, Basic Books, 1958. https://archive.org/details/currentconcepts00jaho
16 Parloff MB, Kelman HC, Frank JD: Comfort, effectiveness, and self-awareness as criteria of improvement in psychotherapy. Am J Psychiatry 1954;11:343–351.
17 Ellis A, Becker I: A Guide to Personal Happiness. Hollywood, Melvin Powers Wilshire Book Company, 1982.
18 Fordyce MW: A program to increase happiness. J Couns Psychol 1983;30:483–498.
19 Padesky CA: Schema change processes in cognitive therapy. Clin Psychol Psychother 1994;1:267–278.
20 Frisch MB: Quality of life therapy and assessment in health care. Clin Psychol Sci Pract 1998;5:19–40.
21 Horowitz MJ, Kaltreider NB: Brief therapy of stress response syndrome. Psychiatr Clin N Am 1979;2:365–377.

Chapter 2

The Philosophy Student and the Pursuit of a Well-Being-Enhancing Strategy

I was wondering about developing a form of psychotherapy based on psychological well-being, but the idea did not seem to materialize. One day, I evaluated Tom, a 23-year-old philosophy student suffering from a severe form of obsessive-compulsive disorder. The disorder was mainly characterized by obsessions related to his girlfriend Laura and had started about a year before. Since then, Tom was unable to study, did not take any examinations, and stopped going to the university. His social life had also been affected. Aside from Laura, whom he kept on pestering with questions about her past, he stopped seeing friends. Tom went to see a psychiatrist, who prescribed fluvoxamine, a selective serotonin reuptake inhibitor. However, the medication did not yield any relief and the psychiatrist switched him to clomipramine, a tricyclic antidepressant drug. Yet, again, no response was observed. These medications were reasonable and appropriate prescriptions on the basis of the available literature. He then underwent cognitive behavior therapy (CBT), but he dropped out of treatment after 6 sessions because he felt he was getting worse. The latter event attracted my attention.

Generally, in the clinical literature no response and deterioration are considered to be the same thing. Yet they are different. In the 1990s, a group of Yale investigators headed by Ralph Horwitz [1] reanalyzed the data of a larger randomized controlled trial that involved the use of a β-blocker after myocardial infarction. Randomized controlled trials are not intended to answer questions about the treatment of individual patients, but to compare the efficacy of a treatment for the average patient who is randomly assigned to one of the groups. Horwitz et al. [1] analyzed the trial in a different way, according to subgroups characterized by specific clinical histories. They found that the β-blocker was helpful for the 'average' patient who survived an acute myocardial infarction, whereas it was harmful in a subgroup characterized by specific cotherapy histories.

If we accept the possibility that a treatment which is helpful on average may be ineffective in some cases and even harmful in someone else, we may learn that a given therapy may not be of value for a particular class or subgroup of subjects who present with certain clinical characteristics [1]. Big Pharma, which together with biotechnology corporations substantially controls medical publications and information [2], does not like to hear about the subgroup which gets worse, probably because it may scare potential customers. Yet these events occur with any drug. I have studied the paradoxical reactions that may take place with antidepressant drugs (when medications deepen the depressed mood) [3]. Clinical worsening may also occur with psychotherapy. The various psychotherapy schools also do not like to hear about negative effects [4].

In clinical pharmacology, adverse events may be due to the fact that the physician did not prescribe the drug appropriately (e.g., at a dosage that is excessive or inadequate); however, in this case treatment was correct. In psychotherapy, negative effects may arise because of psychotherapy that is not properly conducted [4]. However, in the case of Tom, I knew the psychologist who used CBT and held him in high regard for his competence and skills, particularly in obsessive-compulsive disorder. I thus felt that every reasonable approach had been attempted. What could I do that was different? I thought on the substantial distinction that Tom made: drugs did not help him, while psychotherapy made him worse.

I formulated a hypothesis. The basic mechanism of cognitive therapy lies in monitoring distress: identification of the situations where it occurs leads to finding the negative thinking (automatic thoughts) that is associated and precedes the negative emotions (fig. 1). Yet, in the case of Tom, this mechanism probably leads to deepening of distress. What about doing the opposite: monitoring well-being and looking at what interrupts it (fig. 2)? So I told Tom that he had to keep a diary where he should report the instances of well-being. I did not provide any definition of well-being, but I asked him to write down the situations when he felt good, what he experienced, and its intensity. His comment was not encouraging: 'It will be a blank diary.'

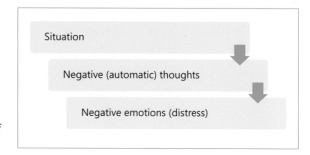

Fig. 1. Basic mechanism of cognitive therapy.

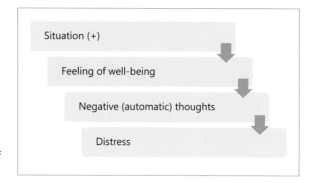

Fig. 2. Basic mechanism of Well-Being Therapy.

Second Session

When he came back, he had his diary. He had written a few instances of well-being. He reluctantly acknowledged that they were present, but added 'they were extremely short, a few minutes only'. Table 1 illustrates one of these instances. I was surprised to see that, even in the midst of distress and suffering, there were some good times, although they were brief. Tom was then instructed to report also which thoughts led to a premature interruption of these instances of well-being. Again I did not share with him information about the type of thoughts we were looking for (automatic thoughts) and the potential explanations that could be made. I wanted him to develop his own antidote.

I did, however, write down in his diary a few things (I always write in the diaries of my patients: instructions for taking medications, behavioral assignments, things we discussed in the session that I feel important). I asked him to go back to the university every other day and to select one exam to be taken. He

Table 1. Second session

Situation	Feeling of well-being	Intensity (0 – 100)
Late afternoon. I am at home studying. Laura will be coming soon.	I am happy to see her.	40

complained, 'It makes no sense. I am no longer able to study.' I replied that gradually we would have come back to it, and I shared with him the story of when I broke my leg while skiing at the age of 11. It was a bad fracture and the orthopedic surgeon applied a cast. I had to keep it for three and a half months, without ever standing up. Finally the day came when my cast had to be taken off, and I thought my agony would be over. My parents did not tell me anything; I thought that my bone had been fixed and I could get up and run. When the surgeon removed the cast, I discovered it was not true at all: my leg had no muscle, I could not bend the knee and when I tried to stand up I realized I was not able to. I started crying, saying that my life was ruined and that I could no longer walk. I do not know whether the clinical choice of the surgeon had been the best also in those days, but his response was:

> Do not cry, Giovanni. It is the way it should be. Now you should start doing some exercise [he just gave me a couple of hints; there was no physical therapy in the place where I lived]. But remember: some days you will feel that you are making progress, that you can bend your knee a little more than the previous days. Other days, you will feel that it is getting worse, that you bend your knee less. Do not worry. Keep on doing what I told you. You will run again.

This is what happened and I often share this story with patients. Therapist self-disclosure was found in psychotherapy research to lower patient distress [5], and I have always felt that it is important for a physician to transmit both technical and emotional knowledge.

Third Session

Tom came back 2 weeks later with his diary. Table 2 displays one example of the situations he wrote.

Table 2. Third session

Situation	Feeling of well-being	Interrupting thoughts
Morning. I am at home studying.	I was able to study well for one entire hour.	Now something will happen to spoil your morning → obsession.

I must say that I did not know what to expect. Tom was a bright, well-educated, and sensitive young man. I wanted to see whether, with some simple indications (as my orthopedic surgeon), he could develop his way to recovery. Indeed he had identified not only feelings of well-being, but what interrupted those feelings. I was using the framework of rationale-emotive and cognitive therapies, and I decided then to opt for the cognitive schema. I thus explained to him what automatic thoughts are [6]. I used Aaron Beck's description [6]. They often occur in specific situations and do not arise as a result of reasoning or reflection, but by reflex. They are relatively autonomous: the subject makes no effort to initiate them and often has troubles turning them off [6]. I explained to Tom how some thoughts he had reported could fit Beck's model of automatic thought [6]. I then asked him to add another column to his diary (in addition to situation, feeling of well-being, and interrupting thoughts) that was indicated as 'observer's interpretation'; in this column he should write what an observer (actually the subject distancing himself/herself from the situation) would be likely to think in those circumstances. At the same time I continued to write behavioral prescriptions in the diary. In addition to attending the university again, he had selected the topic of a course he had already attended for a potential exam. I asked him to attempt to study again, with increasing times of application (15 min first, then 30 min, then 1 h, and so on). He was asked to come back in 2 weeks.

Fourth Session

Tom showed me his diary. He reported several instances of being able to practice self-observation of well-being, to establish a relation between interruption of well-being and thoughts, and to challenge his assumptions, demonstrating that these assumptions were not correct. Two examples are reported in table 3.

Table 3. Fourth session

Situation	Feeling of well-being	Interrupting thoughts	Observer's interpretation
Afternoon. I am going to the supermarket.	I feel calm and relaxed. It is a beautiful day.	I do not deserve these feelings. I cannot feel good. My life is miserable → obsessions.	It is obvious you feel good. There is nothing special in what you are doing.
Morning. I am at home studying.	I am working well this morning.	I am doing this only because I forget my turmoil inside.	There is no turmoil inside, only thoughts. You are not worried about the turmoil, you seek distress.

I was particularly impressed by what he wrote in the observer's interpretation of the second situation: 'you seek distress'. I had the perception that people like him had a low tolerance for well-being and promptly develop thoughts that may lead them back to distress, the condition that they ultimately believe they deserve. I thought of the patient I had seen with George Engel and his description of 'pain-prone personalities' [7].

I thought of my high school studies in Italy. I had attended, like Tom, a 'classic lyceum' where Latin, ancient Greek, and philosophy were the main subjects. I was not particularly fond of Latin and Greek (why did we not study English?), but I have to admit that they provided a unique background. A Greek notion was that if things go very well, the gods may become envious and strike you. In many literary situations it was clear that this was because success can make you underestimate the situations, feel invulnerable, and force you into major mistakes. In other words, one can make gross mistakes at the top of success that would not be made before climbing the ladder (there are almost daily examples of these phenomena with politicians, actors, etc.). Other people, however, are not carried out by these feelings of well-being and indeed are convinced that their success cannot last. I also thought of the Roman philosopher Seneca and his idea that well-being was a learning process and that writing could be instrumental.

At this point I was curious to see what Tom would develop for the next time period. I praised his work and encouraged him to come back with more mate-

Table 4. Sixth session

Situation	Feeling of well-being	Interrupting thoughts	Observer's interpretation
Morning. At home studying.	I have been able to understand a very difficult part of the exam. I am in good shape.	Now I will get stuck in something else and my obsessions will start.	You can control this. The problem is that you got used to obsession, you are anxious and not having them creates anxiety. So you look for them. But the contrast that today is difficult, will be easier and easier.
Evening. At home. The bell is ringing. It is Laura.	Finally! I was really looking forward to seeing her.	Now my obsessions will start and spoil my evening.	You are so damned scared of something spoiling your well-being that you are calling for it. Get used to feeling well!

rial. I also encouraged him to dedicate more time to studying and social activities. There was a clear-cut decrease in his obsessions: they had become less frequent and less intense.

Fifth to Seventh Sessions

The fifth session was also concerned with discussion of the material he had brought with him. In some instances he was unable to provide a valid observer's interpretation and I had to add it. In other cases, what he wrote was fascinating. The time he was able to concentrate was progressively increasing and he had made a tentative plan for an examination. By analyzing the material with him, I had also become aware that some impairments in the psychological well-being dimensions elaborated by Marie Jahoda [8] and Carol Ryff [9] were present and I started discussing them with him. I decided to see him again in a month, to give him more time to progress on his own. The sixth session was very rich with material (a sample is included in table 4).

His observer's interpretations were increasing and rich in philosophical quotations. I explained to him, however, that the diary was not an intellectual exer-

Table 5. Last session

Situation	Feeling of well-being	Interrupting thoughts	Observer's interpretation
Morning. At the university.	I feel very optimistic about my future and my relationship with Laura.	Everything got better very fast; there should be a trick somewhere.	Happiness does not harm. It is silly to be worried about it. If you have the right attitude, you may build it up. And you are getting the right attitude.
Afternoon. I got a very good grade at the university.	Things are really looking up.	My obsessions will come back and I'll be back where I started.	Anxiety makes you see things that do not exist. You see them because you are afraid of them. The more you fear anxiety and its manifestations, the more anxiety gets power. But you have learned how to win.

cise that had to be performed after the events. It could be used 'in vivo' while experiencing the interruption of well-being, as a way of preventing the obsessions. The obsessions continued to decrease in their frequency, intensity, and in their invalidating impact. I had not applied any cognitive restructuring directed to the obsessive thoughts, only to the thoughts interrupting well-being. I gave Tom an appointment in another month. In the interval he passed an exam very well and immediately started planning another one. After the seventh session, I decided that the end of our therapy was approaching, even though I remained a little skeptical about the stability of the results and was reluctant to see what happened as a therapeutic success. Could this be due to my Greek studies?

Eighth and Last Session

After 1 month, Tom came back. It was difficult to recognize the student I had first encountered. He brought his diary (a couple of examples are outlined in table 5). We discussed how he had got rid of most of his obsessions; his life was changing, he was progressing well to a college degree and he was making plans for studies outside the realms of philosophy. In the seventh session I had introduced the idea of closing therapy (I must say that at the beginning of our encounters, because of the novelty of my approach, we had not agreed upon a specific number of sessions). I asked him whether he was ready to go on by himself. He said yes with a lot of determination. I told him, as I always do with my patients, that in any case, for any reason, I was there. He could call me or come to see me. Nonetheless, I wanted to see him in a year to check his progress. I expressed my sincere gratitude to him for the things I had learned through our encounter. One year later, he was fine and had just started a Master's course in marketing – Tom confided 'too much philosophy is not good for me'. I am very proud of him and of his subsequent accomplishments in life.

Posttherapy Reflections

Soon after the therapy was over, I started wondering what had actually happened. I remember one day in Albuquerque I was discussing a case with a resident in psychiatry and my mentor Robert Kellner during the weekly meeting of our psychiatric unit. A patient was not responding to treatment and I had decided to switch her from one drug to another. She had improved very much and rapidly, and I suggested a possible neurotransmitter mechanism for it. The resident had a different view in terms of receptor modifications and we started a lively discussion.

We did not notice that a nurse was trying to say something, unsuccessfully. But during a pause of our debate she said, 'I do not know how to tell you this, docs. But the truth is that we forgot to change the medication and the patient is still taking the old one.' I wished I could have magically disappeared from the room. I was so ashamed of myself and of our silly discussion. But Robert Kellner was, as always, very kind and supportive and explained:

> This case offers a very good lesson. When a patient gets better, the most likely explanation and the one you should keep in mind is that this has nothing to do with what you did, prescribed, or said. There are many potential explanations you may not be even aware of. Only controlled studies may ascertain whether there is something therapeutic in what you are doing.

So my first reaction was: who knows what made Tom get better? Maybe it was the quality of our relationship, my stories, or something that happened to him in the course of therapy. I had found a road to recovery that was not the usual one, but I needed to test it in a scientific way.

References

1 Horwitz RI, Singer BH, Makuch RW, Viscoli CM: Can treatment that is helpful on average be harmful to some patients? J Clin Epidemiol 1996;49:395–400.

2 Abramson J: Overdosed America. New York, Harper, 2005.

3 Fava GA: Do antidepressant and antianxiety drugs increase chronicity in affective disorders? Psychother Psychosom 1994;61:125–131.

4 Linden M: How to define, find and classify side effects in psychotherapy. Clin Psychol Psychother 2013;20:286–296.

5 Barrett MS, Berman J: Is psychotherapy more effective when therapists disclose information about themselves? J Consult Clin Psychol 2001;69:597–603.

6 Beck AT: Cognitive Therapy and the Emotional Disorders. New York, International Universities Press, 1976.

7 Engel GL: 'Psychogenic' pain and the pain-prone patient. Am J Med 1959;26:899–918.

8 Jahoda M: Current Concepts of Positive Mental Health. New York, Basic Books, 1958.

9 Ryff CD: Happiness is everything, or is it? Explorations on the meaning of psychological well-being. J Pers Soc Psychol 1989;6:1069–1081.

Chapter 3

The Process of Validation of Well-Being Therapy

After finding a well-being-enhancing strategy, I realized that several steps were necessary to go further. Even though the first case involved a case of an acute invalidating obsessive-compulsive disorder, the area where I wanted to apply these methods was the residual phase of mood and anxiety disorders, particularly as to relapse prevention. The methodology that I needed to use had to be that of controlled investigations, as Robert Kellner had taught me. I had to involve my research group, i.e., the people who had believed in me and in my odd ideas.

A characteristic of the studies I am going to describe is that they did not involve large populations (in Italy research funding is minimal), but were very careful in assessment and methodology. I personally knew each patient who was involved. The data were expressed by numbers, but I had in mind the actual patients, their faces, and our encounters. The first question was whether patients who were judged to be remitted upon pharmacological and/or psychological treatment from their mood or anxiety disorders displayed less well-being compared to healthy controls who were never ill.

Carol Ryff [1] had developed a questionnaire, the Psychological Well-Being Scales (PWB) for measuring psychological well-being. In those years, however, there was no information as to its application to clinical populations. I thus decided to perform a controlled comparison between a small group of patients we defined as cured and a control group. We used, in addition to the self-rating PWB, a scale that involves a semistructured research interview, the Clinical Interview for Depression (CID) [2]. It offers a very accurate exploration of depressive and anxiety symptoms and is probably the best instrument that is available. It has not been used as much as it should be in research because it takes more time than other scales. A third instrument that we employed was a very brief self-rating questionnaire developed by Robert Kellner, the Symptom Questionnaire (SQ) [3]. It covers both distress and well-being. The well-being scales reflect psychological states (relaxation, contentment, physical well-being, and friendliness), which are quite different from the dimensions of PWB. We found these assessment methods very helpful in other studies we performed. Remitted patients displayed significantly more symptoms than healthy controls, as expected. But they also showed significant impairments in all areas of psychological well-being covered by the PWB [4]. I realized that these patients were better, but not well.

Gratified by the degree of improvement that I had observed in these patients, I forgot that there were still problems. This situation was ideal for testing my psychotherapeutic strategy. I formulated a treatment protocol that was in part based on my experience with Tom, where the articulation of each session was specified, and called it 'Well-Being Therapy (WBT)' [5]. We had developed a certain experience with cognitive behavior treatment (CBT) of residual symptoms of depression, which was found to be more effective than a control condition [6], and I thought that comparing the two strategies (CBT and WBT) could be the first step.

Twenty patients with affective disorders [major depression, panic disorder with agoraphobia, social phobia, generalized anxiety disorder (GAD), obsessive-compulsive disorder] who had been successfully treated by behavioral (anxiety disorders) or pharmacological (mood disorders) methods were randomly assigned to either WBT or CBT for residual symptoms [7]. Both WBT and CBT were associated with a significant reduction of residual symptoms as measured by the CID [2] and in PWB well-being [1]. However, when residual symptoms of the two groups were compared after treatment, a significant advantage of WBT over CBT was observed with the CID. WBT was also associated with a significant increase in PWB well-being, particularly in the personal growth scale. The small number of subjects suggested caution in interpreting this difference and the need for further studies with larger samples of patients with specific mood or anxiety disorders.

These preliminary results pointed to the feasibility of WBT in the residual stage of these disturbances. The improvement in residual symptoms may be explained on the basis of the balance between positive and negative affect [7]. If treatment of psychiatric symptoms induces improvement of well-being – and indeed subscales describing well-being are more sensitive to drug effects than subscales describing symptoms [3] – it is conceivable that changes in well-being may affect the balance of positive and negative affect. In this sense, the higher degree of symptomatic improvement that was observed with WBT in this study is not surprising: in the acute phase of affective illness, removal of symptoms may yield the most substantial changes, but the reverse may be true in its residual phase.

The Big Challenge

As other investigators in the field of depression, I was particularly concerned about the high risk of relapse [8]. It was not easy to make the patients better, but it was even more difficult to keep them well. We had performed a small controlled study on the effects of addressing residual symptomatology with cognitive behavioral methods on relapse rates. Compared to a control condition, there were significant differences after 4 years [9], but not after 6 years [10]. I felt that what I had introduced (a sequential strategy: first treatment with antidepressant drugs and then CBT of residual symptoms) was good, but it was not sufficient. I wanted to repeat the study in patients with a severe form of recurrent depression defined as the occurrence of three or more episodes of unipolar depression, with the immediately preceding episode being no more than 2.5 years before the onset of the current episode [11]. This time, however, I wanted to include WBT in the treatment package, together with cognitive behavior treatment of residual symptoms and lifestyle modification. Forty patients with recurrent major depression, who had been successfully treated with antidepressant drugs, were randomly assigned to either this package including WBT or clinical management. In clinical management, the same number of sessions that was used in the experimental condition was given. Clinical management consisted of reviewing the patient's clinical status and providing the patient with support and advice, if necessary. Specific interventions such as exposure strategies, diary work, and cognitive restructuring were proscribed. The scope was to compare the experimental condition with a group that receives the nonspecific therapeutic ingredients shared by most forms of psychotherapy (table 1) [12, 13].

Table 1. Nonspecific therapeutic ingredients common to most forms of psychotherapy

	Ingredient	Characteristics
1	Attention	The therapist's full availability for specific times
2	Disclosure	The patient's opportunity to share thoughts and feelings
3	High arousal	An emotionally charged, confiding relationship with a helping person
4	Interpretation	A plausible explanation for the patient's problems and difficulties
5	Rituals	A procedure that requires the active participation of both patient and therapist

In both groups, antidepressant drugs were tapered and discontinued. The group that received CBT and WBT had a significantly lower level of residual symptoms after drug discontinuation in comparison with the clinical management group. CBT also resulted in a significantly lower relapse rate (25%) at a 2-year follow-up than did clinical management (80%). At the 6-year follow-up [14], the relapse rate was 40% in the former group and 90% in the latter. Further, the group treated with CBT and WBT had a significantly lower number of recurrences when multiple relapses were taken into account. Even though it was a small and preliminary study, the results were quite impressive: more than half of the patients treated with CBT and WBT were well and drug-free at the 6-year follow-up [14].

The findings were replicated by three independent studies. In a multicenter trial performed in Germany, 180 patients with three or more episodes of major depression were randomized to a combination of CBT, WBT, and mindfulness-based cognitive therapy, or to manualized psychoeducation [15]. Even though the follow-up was limited to 1 year (in our study the most substantial differences emerged later) and medication was continued, there was a significant effect of the experimental condition on the relapse rate of the patients with a high risk of recurrence.

In the United States, Kennard et al. [16] applied the sequential treatment we had introduced in adults [11] to 144 children and adolescents with major depression. They were treated with fluoxetine for 6 weeks, and those who displayed an adequate response were randomized to receive continued medication management or CBT to address residual symptoms and WBT in addition to fluoxetine. The CBT/WBT combination was effective in reducing the risk of relapse, a finding that was quite exceptional in the literature concerned with children and adolescents with major depression. Unfortunately, unlike in our original study [11], medication was continued also in the CBT/WBT group, despite the problems that are related to long-term treatment with antidepressant drugs in that patient population [17].

A third confirmation came from an Iranian study by Moeenizadeh and Salagame [18]. Forty high school and university students suffering from depression were randomly assigned to WBT or CBT. The results unequivocally showed that WBT was more effective than CBT in improving symptoms of depression [18]. The severity of the depressive disturbances was not specifically evaluated and the symptomatology was probably mild. Nonetheless, the results were quite impressive.

Understanding the Specificity of Well-Being Therapy

My research group was very pleased with the results obtained with our approach to recurrent depression [11, 14]. In discussing the data with Chiara Rafanelli, who had performed all psychological evaluations blind to the treatment assignments, an important issue came up. What was the specific role of WBT? In our previous study that did not involve WBT [6, 9, 10], the results had been less positive, but this did not necessarily mean that WBT was responsible for them.

Chiara Rafanelli and I thus decided to perform another controlled investigation. The object of our study this time was a very common form of anxiety, GAD. We had come to the conclusion that probably the sequential combination of CBT and WBT was our best bet in an acute disorder, but was this combination going to be better than just performing CBT? Twenty patients with GAD were randomly assigned to 8 sessions of CBT or the sequential administration of CBT followed by another 4 sessions of WBT [19]. Both treatments were associated with a significant reduction of anxiety. However, significant advantages of the CBT/WBT sequential combination over CBT were observed, both in terms of symptom reduction and psychological well-being improvement as measured by CID [2], PWB [1], and SQ [3]. These results suggested the feasibility and clinical advantages of adding WBT to the treatment of GAD. A possible explanation of these findings is that self-monitoring of episodes of well-being may lead to a more comprehensive identification of automatic thoughts than that entailed by the customary monitoring of episodes of distress in cognitive therapy [20], and therefore may result in more effective cognitive restructuring. These results also lend support to our hypothesis that WBT provides something that CBT alone does not possess.

Addressing Cyclothymic Disorder

Until then we had conceptualized WBT essentially as a tool for increasing psychological well-being in people who had impaired levels. But in my clinical practice I had observed patients in whom these psychological dimensions were exaggerated or unrealistic, whose environmental mastery, for instance, led them to take too many challenges and to be under very stressful situations. Was the role of WBT simply that of a well-being enhancer or could it also serve a stabilizing function?

We thus decided to apply WBT to treatment of cyclothymic disorder, which involves mild or moderate fluctuations of mood, thought, and behavior without meeting formal diagnostic criteria for either major depressive disorder or mania [21]. It is a common and disabling condition that does not attract much research attention since no drugs have been patented for its treatment. Sixty-two patients with cyclothymic disorder were randomly assigned to the sequential combination of CBT and WBT or clinical management. An independent blind evaluator assessed the patients before treatment, after therapy, and at 1- and 2-year follow-ups. The CID [2] and the Mania Scale developed by Per Bech and his collaborators [22] were used to evaluate symptoms. After treatment, a significant difference was found in outcome measures, with greater improvements in the CBT/WBT group compared to clinical management. Therapeutic gains were maintained at the 1- and 2-year follow-ups [21]. The results thus indicate that WBT may address both polarities of mood swings and comorbid anxiety, and may yield significant and lasting benefits in cyclothymic disorder.

What Is the Role of Well-Being Therapy?

The studies that are summarized in this chapter and other investigations that are going to be discussed later in this book indicate that WBT's potential role was broader than originally assumed (improving the risk of relapse in the residual phase of mood and anxiety disorders). Developing the protocols for these studies and using WBT in clinical practice paved the way for a refinement of the original formulation of WBT [5]. With the contribution of Elena Tomba, a first modification was offered in 2009 [23]. Further input came when a leading figure of American CBT, Jesse H. Wright, started using WBT [24]. In Part II of this book, I will describe how WBT can actually be implemented in clinical practice. After a chapter on clinical evaluation, the 8-session program will be described. Such a format, when needed, can be extended to 12 or more sessions or abridged to 4 sessions if preceded by CBT.

References

1 Ryff CD: Psychological well-being revisited. Psychother Psychosom 2014;83:10–28.
2 Guidi J, Fava GA, Bech P, Paykel ES: The Clinical Interview for Depression: a comprehensive review of studies and clinimetric properties. Psychother Psychosom 2011;80: 10–27.
3 Kellner R: A symptom questionnaire. J Clin Psychiatry 1987;48:268–274.
4 Rafanelli C, Park SK, Ruini C, Ottolini F, Cazzaro M, Grandi S, Fava GA: Rating well-being and distress. Stress Med 2000;16:55–61.
5 Fava GA: Well-being therapy: conceptual and technical issues: Psychother Psychosom 1999; 68:171–179.
6 Fava GA, Grandi S, Zielezny M, Canestrari R, Morphy MA: Cognitive behavioral treatment of residual symptoms in primary major depressive disorder. Am J Psychiatry 1994;151: 1295–1299.
7 Fava GA, Rafanelli C, Cazzaro M, Conti S, Grandi S: Well-being therapy: a novel psychotherapeutic approach for residual symptoms of affective disorders. Psychol Med 1998;28:475–480.
8 Fava GA: The concept of recovery in affective disorders. Psychother Psychosom 1996;65: 2–13.
9 Fava GA, Grandi S, Zielezny M, Rafanelli C, Canestrari R: Four-year outcome for cognitive behavioral treatment of residual symptoms in major depression. Am J Psychiatry 1996;153:945–947.

10 Fava GA, Ruini C, Rafanelli C, Finos L, Conti S, Grandi S: Six-year outcome of cognitive behavior therapy for prevention of recurrent depression. Am J Psychiatry 1998,161:1872–1876.
11 Fava GA, Rafanelli C, Grandi S, Conti S, Belluardo P: Prevention of recurrent depression with cognitive behavioral therapy: preliminary findings. Arch Gen Psychiatry 1998;55: 816–820.
12 Frank JD, Frank B: Persuasion and Healing. Baltimore, Johns Hopkins University Press, 1991.
13 Fava GA, Sonino N: Psychosomatic medicine. Int J Clin Practice 2010;64:999–1001.
14 Fava GA, Ruini C, Rafanelli C, Finos L, Conti S, Grandi S: Six-year outcome of cognitive behavior therapy for prevention of recurrent depression. Am J Psychiatry 2004;161:1872–1876.
15 Stangier U, Hilling C, Heidenreich T, Risch AK, Barocka A, Schlösser R, Kronfeld K, Ruckes C, Berger H, Röschke J, Weck F, Volk S, Hambrecht M, Serfling R, Erkwoh R, Stirn A, Sobanski T, Hautzinger M: Maintenance cognitive-behavioral therapy and manualized psychoeducation in the treatment of recurrent depression: a multicenter prospective randomized controlled trial. Am J Psychiatry 2013;170:624–632.

16 Kennard BD, Emslie GJ, Mayes TL, Nakonezny PA, Jones JM, Foxwell AA, King J: Sequential treatment with fluoxetine and relapse-prevention CBT to improve outcomes in pediatric depression. Am J Psychiatry 2014;171:1083–1090.

17 Offidani E, Fava GA, Sonino N: Iatrogenic comorbidity in childhood and adolescence: new insights from the use of antidepressant drugs. CNS Drugs 2014;28:769–774.

18 Moeenizadeh M, Salagame KKK: The impact of well-being therapy on symptoms of depression. Int J Psychol Stud 2010;2:223–230.

19 Fava GA, Ruini C, Rafanelli C, Finos L, Salmaso L, Mangelli L, Sirigatti S: Well-being therapy of generalized anxiety disorder. Psychother Psychosom 2005;74:26–30.

20 Beck AT, Emery G: Anxiety Disorders and Phobias. Cambridge, Basic Books, 1985.

21 Fava GA, Rafanelli C, Tomba E, Guidi J, Grandi S: The sequential combination of cognitive behavioral treatment and well-being therapy in cyclothymic disorder. Psychother Psychosom 2011;80:136–143.

22 Bech P, Kastrup M, Rafaelsen OJ: Mini-compendium of rating scales for states of anxiety, depression, mania, schizophrenia with corresponding DSM-III syndromes. Acta Psychiatr Scand 1986;73(suppl 326):1–37

23 Fava GA, Tomba E: Increasing psychological well-being and resilience by psychotherapeutic methods. J Pers 2009;77:1903–1934.

24 Wright JH, McCray LW: Breaking Free from Depression. Pathways to Wellness. New York, Guilford Press, 2012.

Chapter 4
Initial Evaluation

The scope of the initial evaluation is to assess the feasibility of Well-Being Therapy (WBT) in a specific case. In the past two decades, an oversimplified and reductionist approach in clinical medicine, subsumed under the rubric of evidence-based medicine, has produced the following logical sequence. It is important to get a diagnosis; if a certain type of treatment (e.g., a medication) has been found to be effective in randomized controlled trials (summarized by statistical procedures known as meta-analyses), it should be applied [1]. As Healy [2, p. 200] remarked:

> …randomized placebo-controlled trials originated as an effort to debunk therapeutic claims, but the force field in which medicine is now practiced has transformed them in technologies that mandate action… Where the placebo arms of antidepressant, antipsychotic or mood stabilizer trials suggest we should not be using the drugs as readily as we do, the trials of these products, embodied in guidelines, have instead become a means to enforce treatment.

Probably as a reaction to the pharmaceutical drive to universal consumption of psychotropic drugs, psychotherapy has followed a similar route. If a psychotherapeutic approach has been found to be effective in a specific diagnostic group (e.g., panic disorder), it should be applied. This line of reasoning forgets the fact that no treatment is effective in 100% of cases, and that it may even be counterproductive in some instances, as discussed in Chapter 2. Cognitive behavior therapy (CBT) has certainly been found to be highly effective in panic disorder [3], but, as a clinician, I would not suggest it to every patient with panic. My decision would depend on a broader assessment rooted in clinical thinking.

Chiara Rafanelli, Elena Tomba, and I have discussed how the mere psychiatric diagnosis, as formulated in *Diagnostic and Statistical Manual of Mental Disorders* (DSM) [4], is not sufficient to articulate the clinical process [5]. First of all, exclusive reliance on a limited range of symptoms and the resulting diagnostic criteria has impoverished the clinical process and does not reflect the complex thinking that underlies decisions in psychiatric practice [5]. We need a much broader range of information, encompassing stress, lifestyle, subclinical symptoms, illness behavior, psychological well-being, interpersonal relationships, and social support [6].

Second, we need to organize these clinical data in a comprehensive framework for clinical reasoning [6]. We have suggested the usefulness of a framework developed by Paul Emmelkamp (Professor of Clinical Psychology at the University of Amsterdam) and his group – macroanalysis [7]. It consists of establishing a relationship between co-occurring syndromes and problems. Macroanalysis is not just limited to diagnostic entities, as the concept of comorbidity in DSM is [5], but also to problems that are judged by the clinician to affect a person's life.

Macroanalysis starts from the assumption that, in most cases, there are functional relationships among different problem areas and that the targets of treatment may vary during the course of the disturbances. Different lines of treatment may be chosen at different times. The hierarchical organization that is chosen may depend on a variety of factors (urgency, availability of treatment tools, priorities established by the clinician and/or the patient, etc.).

For instance, let us consider the case of a depressed patient who meets DSM-5 criteria [4] for a major depressive disorder (fig. 1). The depressive episode, because of the resulting loss of interest and irritability, is causing problems in the family and withdrawal from social activities. Depression is severe and mixed with anxiety symptoms. Macroanalysis helps to identify the main problem areas of this specific situation. Clinical judgment dictates the priority of the interventions. In this case, the most urgent therapeutic decision appears to be the use of antidepressant drugs. Yet, macroanalysis appears to be particularly useful when applied to the longitudinal development of disturbances and their response to treatment. When a new assessment is performed after the first line of treatment (pharmacotherapy) has improved the depressive symptomatology, other areas

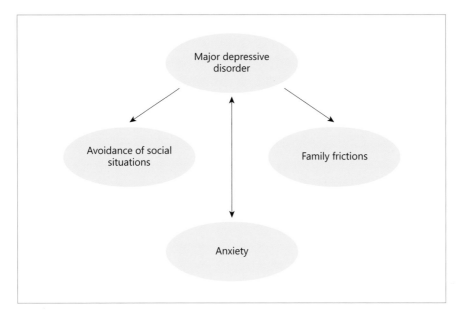

Fig. 1. Macroanalysis of a depressed patient (stage 1).

of concern may emerge (fig. 2). The patient may disclose social phobia and strong feelings of inadequacy that could not be clearly assessed at the time of the first evaluation, in addition to the family problems that had been already identified.

The clinician is thus confronted with three distinct yet ostensibly related problems (fig. 2). He/she may judge these problems to be related to incomplete remission from depression and may increase the medication dose or initiate augmentation strategies. He/she may also decide to address all the problems depicted in figure 2 with a different treatment (e.g., psychotherapy) in a sequential model [5, 8]. Another option would be to tackle one problem at the time, according to a hierarchical line of reasoning. In the case illustrated in figure 2, priority was given to the cognitive behavioral treatment of social phobia. Will treatment of this anxiety disorder result in substantial improvement of feelings of inadequacy and family problems, or will indications for WBT emerge? In this latter case, WBT will supplement CBT. Further examples of the use of macroanalysis may be found in *The Psychosomatic Assessment* [6].

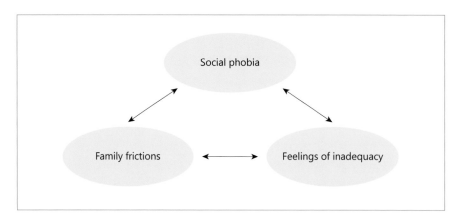

Fig. 2. Macroanalysis of a depressed patient (stage 2).

A third aspect that is crucial in determining the application of a therapeutic approach is concerned with the treatment history of the patient. Elena Tomba [9] observed that under ordinary conditions, patients are included in a trial regardless of their treatment history and defined them as 'nowhere patients'. In the first case where WBT was applied (Chapter 2), treatment history was the variable that led me to attempt a new approach.

Clinicians tend to employ this reasoning in their everyday practice, even though such use is not formally recognized (they may be unaware, for instance, that they are using macroanalysis) and randomized controlled trials apply fixed treatment packages to all patients who are recruited. A relevant exception was the study on WBT in cyclothymic disorder [8] that we discussed in the previous chapter. In that investigation, macroanalysis guided clinical treatment in the experimental group.

WBT should not be used in every patient who meets specific diagnostic criteria as indicated in DSM-5 [4]. It should follow clinical reasoning and case formulation facilitated by the use of macroanalysis. It should be applied to a specific stage of development of a disorder [5], which also includes assessment of treatment responses [9]. The number of sessions should also reflect this line of reasoning.

A question that may arise is whether application of WBT, whether alone or preceded by CBT, requires specific assessment of psychological well-being. We mentioned in the previous chapter two scales, the Psychological Well-Being Scales (PWB) [10] and the Symptom Questionnaire (SQ) [11], which measure different aspects of well-being. There is also a version of the PWB that can be used in a semistructured research interview to increase interaction and feedback from the patient [12]. In our clinical trials, however, therapists were blind to the PWB and SQ scores, and in my practice I have never used them in a systematic way as I generally use the CID [13].

WBT has been found to be effective in depression, generalized anxiety disorder, and cyclothymia, but may potentially be applied to other disorders that are awaiting appropriate testing in controlled trials (we will discuss these potential applications in Part III).

As a general indication, it is difficult to apply WBT as a first-line treatment of an acute psychiatric disorder. It may be more suitable as a second- or third-line treatment. Most of the patients who are seen in clinical practice have complex and chronic disorders [5, 14–16], unlike the symptomatic volunteers who are recruited in the studies, particularly in the US. It is simply wishful thinking (i.e., the oversimplification of evidence-based medicine) to believe that one course of treatment will be sufficient for yielding lasting and satisfactory remission.

In the following chapters, I will outline the 8-session treatment program, keeping in mind that there may be wide variations in its structure and timing, which depend on the purpose and staging of interventions. WBT is a short-term psychotherapeutic strategy that may, when needed, be extended to 12 or more sessions. When it is preceded by CBT, the number of sessions can be abridged to 4 (Chapter 14). The duration of each session may range 40–50 min. The interval between sessions is 2 weeks, but can be shortened to 1 week or extended to longer times if necessary.

References

1 Fava GA, Guidi J, Rafanelli C, Sonino N: The clinical inadequacy of evidence-based medicine and a need for a conceptual framework based on clinical judgment. Psychother Psychosom 2015;84:1–3

2 Healy D: Irrational healers? Psychother Psychosom 2008;77:198–200.

3 Marks IM: Fears, Phobias and Rituals. New York, Oxford University Press, 1987.

4 American Psychiatric Association: Diagnostic and Statistical Manual of Mental Disorders (DSM-5). Arlington, American Psychiatric Association, 2013.

5 Fava GA, Rafanelli C, Tomba E: The clinical process in psychiatry: a clinimetric approach. J Clin Psychiatry 2012;73:177–184.

6 Fava GA, Sonino N, Wise TN (eds): The Psychosomatic Assessment. Basel, Karger, 2012.

7 Emmelkamp PMG, Bouman TK, Scholing A: Anxiety Disorders. Chichester, UK, Wiley, 1993.

8 Fava GA, Rafanelli C, Tomba E, Guidi J, Grandi S: The sequential combination of cognitive behavioral treatment and Well-Being Therapy in cyclothymic disorder. Psychother Psychosom 2011;80:136–143.

9 Tomba E: Nowhere patients. Psychother Psychosom 2012;81:69–72.

10 Ryff CD: Psychological well-being revisited: advances in the science and practice of eudaimonia. Psychother Psychosom 2014;83:10–28.

11 Kellner R: A symptom questionnaire. J Clin Psychiatry 1987;48:268–274.

12 Fava GA, Tomba E: Increasing psychological well-being and resilience by psychotherapeutic methods. J Pers 2009;77:1903–1934.

13 Guidi J, Fava GA, Bech P, Paykel ES: The Clinical Interview for Depression: a comprehensive review of studies and clinimetric properties. Psychother Psychosom 2011;80: 10–27.

14 Vanheule S, Desmet M, Meganck R, Inslegers R, Willemsen J, De Schryver M, Devitsch I: Reliability in psychiatric diagnosis with DSM. Psychother Psychosom 2014;83:313–314.

15 Zimmerman M: Screening for bipolar disorder. Psychother Psychosom 2014;83:259–262.

16 Cosci F, Fava GA: Staging of mental disorders: a systematic review. Psychother Psychosom 2013;82:20–34.

Chapter 5
Session 1

The first session offers the opportunity to become aware of the patient's current problems and past treatment history, which may include both pharmacotherapy and psychotherapy. It is important to get a feeling for previous experiences, successes, and frustrations. This exploration is generally achieved by open-ended questions, with opportunities for clarification, and specific questioning. It is also a chance for the clinician to assess the patient's usual coping behavior. Such initial appraisal does not need to be exhaustive. There will be other opportunities for the patient to share what is going on. The length of this initial phase is variable, but it is necessary to leave at least 15 min for providing an overview of the treatment process. The clinician should be aware that if the patient had received previous evaluations and treatment, almost all the attention would have been dedicated to distress and its consequences. This provides an involuntary but unavoidable reinforcement to the negative aspects of life ('Tell me what is wrong with you. Skip what is going well.'). The change is announced with a statement like this:

> So far we have concentrated on distress and what is wrong with you. The next type of therapy, however, works on your positive part and we try to get rid of what hinders its full development. I am sure we will be able to build on that.

Patients are asked to report in a structured diary the circumstances surrounding their episodes of well-being, rated on a scale from 0 to 100, with 0 being absence of well-being and 100 being the most intense well-being that could be ex-

Table 1. Well-being diary

Situation	Well-being	Intensity[1] (0–100)

[1] 0 indicates the complete absence of well-being, while 100 indicates the most intense well-being that the patient could actually experience.

Table 2. Well-being check

1	My general sense of well-being	_____
2	My sense of well-being as to my physical state	_____
3	Being in charge of the situations in my life	_____
4	My sense of having developed and matured over the years	_____
5	My feeling good about what I can do in the future	_____
6	I am pleased for standing by my principles	_____
7	When I look at the story of my life, I am pleased with how things have turned out	_____
8	My sense of getting a lot from my relationships with others	_____

Please rate your sense of well-being at this point in your life on a scale from 0 to 100 (0 = no sense of well-being; 100 = it could not be better).

perienced (table 1). When patients are assigned this homework, they often object that they will bring a blank diary because they never feel well. It is helpful to reply that these moments do exist but tend to go unnoticed. Patients should therefore monitor them anyway. Jesse Wright and Laura McCray [1] have suggested a 'well-being check-up' that uses a scale from 0 to 100 for rating the overall sense of well-being and well-being in specific areas. It is probably something each of us should be doing from time to time to see how we progress in life. I suggest to use a modified 'well-being check' (table 2). However, this can be performed as an additional assessment tool and is not a part of the homework that is started in table 1.

The patients are also told that the most important part of the therapy is the interval between sessions, i.e., what the patient actually does. There is no a priori explanation of the principles and ideas of Well-Being Therapy (WBT) and

Table 3. Goals of session 1

1	Getting a patient's account of how he/she feels, current and past distress, and treatment history
2	Providing information about the structure and modalities of WBT, including estimated number of sessions, their duration and interval, and expected homework
3	Establishing a first communication channel and building the basis of a therapeutic alliance
4	Introducing the concept of self-therapy
5	Giving a first homework assignment (the well-being diary)

not even of what we mean by well-being. This will emerge in due course. It is just specified that we mean both experiences and feelings. If we want to free the patient's strengths, we cannot use structures that are too rigid and predetermined. We need to explore each individual's unique universe and meanings.

The clinician closes the session by introducing the concept of self-therapy:

If the doctor finds that you have high cholesterol, he/she may prescribe a medication to lower your cholesterol. But your doctor will also give you some advice about what is good for you (e.g., certain types of food, physical exercise) and what is bad (e.g., high cholesterol food, inactivity, smoking). This self-therapy is at least as important as medication. Our self-therapy is not that simple, but follows the same principles.

The patient is thus asked to use the assessment diary for the 2-week period before the next session, and the clinician should explain: 'It is our first step together. It is so important. You do not need to write every day or long reports. I do not care about style. But I really look forward to reading it.' Table 3 summarizes the goals of the session.

References

1 Wright JH, McCray LW: Breaking Free from Depression. Pathways to Wellness. New York, Guilford Press, 2012.

Chapter 6
Session 2

When the patient comes back, a wide range of possibilities occur. The most favorable is that the patient has brought back the diary or at least has scribbled a few things on a piece of paper. I personally emphasize the importance of traditional writing and I discourage the use of computer-assisted homework, but this is a limitation of mine that younger therapists performing Well-Being Therapy do not have. If material is presented, I commend the patient before examining it, just as a matter of principle. If no material is brought, I dedicate the session to exploring the current situation, resistances, difficulties, and misunderstandings, and I clearly tell the patient that we are stuck until self-therapy begins.

In developing this protocol I was influenced by my experience with behavioral treatment of phobic disorders, particularly panic disorder with agoraphobia [1] and social phobia [2]. By using homework assignments in treating patients, I learned how important it is to move very gradually, but in a progressive way, and not to mix cognitive restructuring and exposure from the beginning (I will discuss these strategies in Chapter 17). Monitoring experiences and feelings of well-being introduces the patient to self-observation, which is a therapeutic ingredient [3].

Meehl [4] described 'how people with low hedonic capacity should pay greater attention to the "hedonic book keeping" of their activities than would be necessary for people located midway or high on the hedonic capacity continuum.

Table 1. Well-being diary of Alex

Situation	Well-being	Intensity (0–100)
I had to deal with a difficult situation at work.	It went better than I thought.	30

That is, it matters more to someone cursed with an inborn hedonic defect whether he is efficient and sagacious in selecting friends, jobs, cities, tasks, hobbies, and activities in general' (p. 305). There has been confirmation of Meehl's observation in two controlled trials [5, 6].

But before discussing the diary with the patient, I want to find out how he/she feels and how things went in the past 2 weeks. I do not want to convey the impression that I am only interested in 'products' (despite my propaganda and praise), and I want to communicate that I am interested in him/her as a person – which is exactly how I feel. By doing this we do not waste time. If the patient is worried about something, his/her concentration is likely to be poor, unless the worry is shared. So we are actually investing in more productive time. A goal of the session is to review the homework.

Generally there are few situations and ratings (0–100), as in the case of the philosophy student I described in Chapter 2 and in the example depicted in table 1. The example involves Alex, a sales person who had to visit a customer who in recent months had complained more and more about products and poor service. Alex was very worried and anxious about visiting him, but things went better than he thought. He felt relieved and when he left the customer was well for a couple of hours.

In this phase it is important to discern and discuss with the patient what led to well-being. First, well-being may simply be a feeling that is a consequence of a break from anxiety and anguish, as in the case of Alex. An issue that is not sufficiently appreciated is the experience of mental pain many patients have [7]. Patients sometimes mention this experience spontaneously; in other cases only upon specific questions (which are, however, seldomly asked). Mental pain may be worse than most forms of physical pain because it is not localized and often has no apparent reason. Table 2 indicates some characteristics of mental pain, as depicted in a self-rating scale. Grief provides an example of the sense of emptiness, loss of meaning, and suffering that mental pain entails. It may or may not

Table 2. The Mental Pain Questionnaire (MPQ; Fava GA)

Mental Pain Questionnaire (MPQ)

Mental or psychological pain is an experience that is part of life. It is different from physical pain. We would like to learn about your experience of mental pain in the past week. There is no right or wrong answer. Please work quickly.

1	I feel pain	Yes	No
2	My heart is broken	Yes	No
3	I will never find again what I have lost	Yes	No
4	My pain is everywhere	Yes	No
5	My pain is with me all the time	Yes	No
6	I cannot understand why I feel this pain	True	False
7	I feel empty	Yes	No
8	My life makes no sense	True	False
9	My pain will never go away	True	False
10	The only way to stop my pain is to die	True	False

be associated with anxiety and/or depression [7]. Well-being may thus result as a break from mental pain. In any event, an important point to explain is that distress is seldom without interruptions and these are the windows of opportunity that we should take advantage of.

Second, well-being may also be related to a particular experience (something the patient does). The term 'pleasant activities' that is used in cognitive therapy may be misleading here. We particularly look for what have been defined as 'optimal' or 'flow' experiences [8]. They are characterized by clear goals, immediate feedback, high challenges matched with adequate personal skills, merging of action and awareness, concentration on the task at hand, perceived control of the situation, loss of self-consciousness, altered sense of time, and intrinsic motivation [8]. Extensive research on the topic has emphasized the perceived match between high challenges and adequate personal skills [9, 10]. The match is dynamic in that the perception of high challenges promotes the increase in related skills. Increased competence, in turn, encourages the individual for more complex challenges that will require higher capabilities [8, 10]. Cross-sectional studies have demonstrated that optimal experience can occur in any daily context, such as work, study, sports, arts, and leisure [10]. Patients are thus asked to report whether they feel optimal experiences in their daily life and are invited to

Table 3. Well-being diary

Situation	Well-being (0–100)	Interfering thoughts or behaviors
Where well-being occurs	Its characteristics and intensity	What leads to termination

Table 4. Goals of session 2

1	Checking how the 2 weeks went for the patient in general
2	Review of the well-being diary and the difficulties related to its completion
3	Beginning to understand which feelings and experiences make the patient feel better
4	Introducing the concept of optimal experiences
5	Introducing monitoring of thoughts and behaviors that interrupt well-being
6	Continuing with homework assignments (well-being diary)

list the associated activities and situations in their diaries. How much time do people devote to these activities? Has this time decreased recently? Patients are then encouraged to look more for optimal experiences and to report them in the diary.

Some attention is also paid to the ratings assigned by the patient to experiences and feelings of well-being. If the ratings are consistently low (e.g., 30), the therapist asks the patient what would potentially represent a rating of 70 or 80. This is done to avoid having the patient focus exclusively on lower levels of well-being. As in the first session, no specific definition of well-being is provided, not the psychological dimensions that characterize it in Jahoda's model [11] and Ryff's questionnaire [12] are introduced.

When scheduling homework exposure to phobic patients, I had to write down the assignments in their diaries. I also began to add sentences that could modulate their behavior ('this was a very good move!', 'you should not have escaped as you did'). Progressively, I wrote in the diary also some issues that we had discussed and that I thought were important. Robert Kellner often reminded me that physicians retain very little from educational activities (often <10%), but are convinced that their patients have 100% recollection of what they were told during a visit. I thus started writing encouragements and subtle behavioral prescriptions in the diary, which I define as 'our diary'.

The patient is asked to continue to use the diary for monitoring well-being, to look for optimal experiences, and report them in a diary. Another appointment is scheduled in 2 weeks. The patient is asked to report more information in the diary, as indicated in table 3. I am interested in what leads to a premature interruption of well-being, either thoughts or behaviors. The main goals of the second session are summarized in table 4.

References

1 Fava GA, Rafanelli C, Grandi S, Conti S, Ruini C, Mangelli L, Belluardo P: Long-term outcome of panic disorder with agoraphobia treated by exposure. Psychol Med 2001;31: 891–898.

2 Fava GA, Grandi S, Rafanelli C, Ruini C, Conti S, Belluardo P: Long-term outcome of social phobia treated by exposure. Psychol Med 2001;31:899–905.

3 Emmelkamp PM: Self-observation versus flooding in the treatment of agoraphobia. Behav Res Ther 1974;12:229–237.

4 Meehl PE: Hedonic capacity: some conjectures. Bull Menninger Clin 1975;39:295–307.

5 Emmons RA, McCullough ME: Counting blessings versus burdens: an experimental investigation of gratitude and subjective well-being in daily life. J Pers Soc Psychol 2003;84: 377–389.

6 Burton CM, King LA: The health benefits of writing about intensely positive experiences. J Res Pers 2004;38:150–163.

7 Tossani E: The concept of mental pain. Psychother Psychosom 2013;82:67–73.

8 Csikszentmihalyi M, Csikszentmihalyi I (eds): Optimal Experience. Psychological Studies of Flow in Consciousness. New York, Cambridge University Press, 1988.

9 Delle Fave A, Fava GA: Positive psychotherapy and social change; in Biswas-Diener R (ed): Positive Psychology as Social Change. New York, Springer, 2011, pp 267–291.

10 Delle Fave A: Past, present, and future of flow; in David SA, Bomwell I, Conley Agers A (eds): The Oxford Handbook of Happiness. Oxford, Oxford University Press, 2013, pp 60–72.

11 Jahoda M: Current Concepts of Positive Mental Health. New York, Basic Books, 1958.

12 Ryff CD: Psychological well-being revisited: advances in the science and practice of eudaimonia. Psychother Psychosom 2014;83:10–28.

Chapter 7

Session 3

This phase of treatment is focused on enhancing the patient's ability to self-monitor periods of well-being and to identify thoughts, beliefs, and behaviors that lead to premature interruption of well-being.

The clinician asks the patient if any difficulty was encountered in completing the homework. If so, troubleshooting is done to identify obstacles to completion. The clinician praises the patient for the work that was completed. For instance, in the case of Alex (described in the previous chapter), some thoughts emerged (table 1).

The similarities with the search for irrational, tension-evoking thoughts in Ellis and Becker's rational-emotive therapy [1] and automatic thoughts in cognitive therapy [2] are obvious. However, the trigger for self-observation is different, being based on well-being instead of distress. Even though techniques derived from rational-emotive therapy can also be employed in Well-Being Therapy (WBT), the cognitive behavioral model has been used in all the studies that have been performed as well as in my own clinical practice [2].

The patient is thus introduced to the concept of automatic thought through examples that may be available in the diary and with additional illustrations. Automatic thoughts can either be a thought or a visual image that the patient may not be aware of unless specific attention is focused on it [2]. They are generally viewed by the individual as factual representations of reality and thus are firmly believed. Automatic thoughts can precede episodes of distress [as monitoring according to the cognitive behavior therapy (CBT) model documents],

Table 1. Well-being diary of Alex

Situation	Well-being (0–100)	Interfering thoughts or behaviors
I had to deal with a difficult situation at work.	It went better than I thought (30).	I was very lucky. But luck cannot last.

but can also lead to interruption of well-being, which may or may not be followed by emergence of distress. Since these cognitions are automatic, habitual, and believable, the individual seldom challenges their validity [2]. Their identification is not an easy job and requires specific practice. Patients should not feel frustrated if they are unable to identify automatic thoughts at the very beginning. If they could easily be caught, they would not be automatic thoughts. This phase is crucial since it allows the therapist to identify which areas of psychological well-being are unaffected by irrational or automatic thoughts and which are saturated with them. The therapist may challenge these thoughts with appropriate questions, such as 'What is the evidence for or against this idea?' or 'Are you thinking in all-or-nothing terms?' [2].

Yet, premature interruption of well-being is not only linked to thoughts and beliefs, but may also be a result of specific behavior. If Alex is convinced (table 1) that the good outcome with the customer was a pure matter of luck, he may decide not to take other risks for that day, to avoid other opportunities that may be challenging at first sight. Alex may decide not to visit other customers that day and by doing this he may miss important opportunities.

In dealing with patients who suffer from agoraphobia, where the individual fears and avoids situations (e.g., public transportation, being in enclosed spaces, or crowds) where escape might be difficult, I realized that these patients limit their exposure to what is essential and unavoidable. Their life may look normal from the outside (e.g., they go to work, they shop), but avoidance puts a subtle constraint on their lives. Similarly, Alex only deals with what is well known and tested. He accurately avoids new situations because he is convinced he cannot make it and that his inadequacy is likely to be disclosed. This requires careful exposure homework, encouraging the patient to meet reasonable challenges, as will be described in the following chapters.

The clinician also takes note of what types of situations/activities may be associated with high pleasure and mastery. Attention is particularly directed to

Table 2. Well-being diary

Situation	Well-being (0–100)	Interfering thoughts or behaviors	Observer

optimal experiences [3, 4]. Massimini and Delle Fave [4] consider optimal experience to be the 'psychic compass' orienting psychological selection (the individual preferential cultivation of a specific set of interests, relations, values, and goals) throughout life. It is not simply a pleasurable experience. It is something that summarizes what an individual has been striving for.

For instance, I have spent my life attempting to find ways to help patients in distress – instead of having fun outside, I have worked hard, reflected on my clinical and life experiences, and spent a lot of time in libraries. By doing this I gave up other things that might have been more pleasurable and less stressful. Yet, the process of writing this book felt like an optimal experience to me: the possibility to transmit a method that may help people makes sense of my efforts. This book was completely handwritten first (there is no other way I can write something that I feel is important) and this probably connects with other earlier experiences. For many years colleagues and coworkers had asked to me to write this book. 'I have no time' was my reply, which was true in a way. However, I could have written fewer articles or scheduled my time in a different way. If writing this book was likely to be an optimal experience, why did I avoid it for so long? Maybe I needed more data, more time, and more experience (and indeed if I had written this book 5 years ago it would have been quite different). The truth, however, was that I did not feel ready or adequate until a magic click in my mind triggered by an apparently casual remark from a colleague made me begin my path.

The clinician should be the trigger for pursuing optimal experiences more actively. The therapist may thus reinforce and encourage activities that are likely to elicit well-being and optimal experiences (e.g., assigning the task of undertaking particular pleasurable activities for a certain time each day). When pleasure is mixed with fear, such reinforcement may also result in graded task assignments [2], with special reference to exposure to feared or challenging

Table 3. Goals of session 3

1	Checking how the 2 weeks went for the patient in general
2	Review of the well-being diary and the difficulties related to its completion
3	Enhancing the understanding of which feelings and experiences make the patient feel better, including optimal experiences
4	Beginning to understand which thoughts and/or behaviors lead to a premature interruption of well-being
5	Introducing the observer's column in the well-being diary
6	Continuing with homework assignments (well-being diary, activities encouragement and scheduling)

situations, which the patient is likely to avoid. The focus of this phase of WBT is always on self-monitoring of moments of feelings of well-being. The therapist, however, refrains from suggesting conceptual and technical alternatives to thoughts that interrupt well-being, or from outlining a graded task assignment, unless a satisfactory degree of self-observation (including irrational or automatic thoughts) has been achieved. Further monitoring is thus requested.

A specific suggestion, which also derives from the CBT model [2], is made: the diary is extended by adding a fourth column that deals with an observer's interpretation, or what another person may think in that situation (table 2). The patient is thus encouraged to develop alternatives to the usual pattern of thinking. The job is not easy since the clinician has not yet provided material that could be helpful in this direction. The goal is simply to increase the level of self-observation. More substantial work will take place in due course.

The patient is asked to come back in 2 weeks with the well-being diary. Table 3 summarizes the main goals of the third session.

References

1 Ellis A, Becker I: *A Guide to Personal Happiness*. Hollywood, Melvin Powers Wilshire Book Company, 1982.
2 Beck AT, Rush AJ, Shaw BF, Emery G: Cognitive Therapy of Depression. New York, Guilford Press, 1979.
3 Csikszentmihalyi M, Csikszentmihalyi I: Optimal Experience. Psychological Studies of Flow in Consciousness. New York, Cambridge University Press, 1988.
4 Massimini F, Delle Fave A: Individual development in a bio-cultural perspective. Am Psychol 2000;55:24–33.

Chapter 8
Session 4

While so far most of the attention has been on monitoring well-being and identifying thoughts and/or behaviors leading to its premature interruption, in this session more substantial work on modifying attitudes toward well-being is pursued.

As before, the clinician first asks how the past 2 weeks went and if any difficulty was encountered in completing the homework. It is emphasized that changes can be achieved but require specific knowledge of what has to be changed, and thus careful monitoring. At this point in treatment, the patient is expected to be able to readily identify moments of well-being (regardless of length), to be aware of interruptions to well-being (thoughts and/or behaviors), and to start wondering whether any alternative thinking or behavior is possible. On the basis of the relatively little information up to this point, the patient generally has difficulties in modifying automatic thoughts and developing alternative interpretations (observer's column).

This is the time when the therapist plays a more active role and adds material for reflections to the well-being diary. After reviewing patient entries in the diary, the clinician begins to work on two converging, yet distinct, paths.

One path is concerned with the standard cognitive behavior therapy work examining the evidence for and against automatic thoughts and definition of thinking errors [1]. The latter include all-or-nothing thinking (all good or all

Table 1. Environmental mastery

Impaired level	Balanced level	Excessive level
The person feels difficulties in managing everyday affairs; he/she feels unable to improve things around; he/she is unaware of opportunities	The person has a sense of competence in managing the environment; he/she makes good use of surrounding opportunities; he/she is able to choose what is more suitable to personal needs	The person is looking for difficult situations to be handled; he/she is unable to savor positive emotions and leisure time; he/she is too engaged in work or family activities

bad), jumping to conclusions (thinking of the worst possible interpretation of the situation), ignoring the evidence (making a judgment without looking at all the information), magnifying or minimizing (magnifying faults or difficulties, and minimizing strengths and opportunities), overgeneralizing (giving a small flaw so much significance that the entire picture is affected), and personalizing (putting oneself at the center of blame and as the cause of failures).

The second path is concerned with attempting to explain the premature interruption of well-being with the help of the dimensions in the framework developed by Marie Jahoda [2] and elaborated by Carol Ryff [3]. The dimensions are introduced as long as the material of the diary lends to their use, and not as a prearranged description. Even when the material may allow discussion of all dimensions, care is exercised in not burdening the patient with an excessive amount of information and no more than two dimensions are discussed in a single session. For simplicity, I will describe in this chapter two dimensions that frequently occur. By no means should these be the first to be discussed. In the following two chapters, I will discuss the other dimensions, but again this does not reflect the actual order they are introduced to the patient, which should be based on the material that is actually presented.

Environmental Mastery (table 1)

This is the most frequent impairment that emerges. It was expressed by Alex as follows: 'I have got a filter that nullifies any positive achievement (I was just lucky) and amplifies any negative outcome, no matter how much expected (this

Table 2. Jahoda's conceptualization of environmental mastery [2]

1	The ability to love
2	Adequacy in love, work, and play
3	Adequacy in interpersonal relationships
4	Readiness to meeting situational requirements
5	Capacity for adaptation and adjustment
6	Efficiency in problem solving

once more confirms I am a failure)' and 'I immediately forget the customers who placed an order. I have in mind only those who did not'. This lack of sense of control leads the patient to miss surrounding opportunities, with the possibility of subsequent regret over them. Environmental mastery is a key mediator or moderator of stressful life experiences. The individual is capable of proactive and effective problem solving, rather than being passively overwhelmed by external forces, but is also capable of finding time for rest and relaxation in daily life [2–4].

While in the initial phase of application of Well-Being Therapy (WBT) I was very concerned with impairments of well-being, I subsequently started noticing, particularly in our work with patients with cyclothymic disorder, that also very high levels of environmental mastery can be dysfunctional (table 1). Individuals may be looking for difficult situations to be handled, engage too much in work, or are totally occupied by family needs and activities. Their abilities in planning and solving problems may lead others to constantly ask for their help, which results in feeling of being exploited and overwhelmed by requests [5]. These attitudes toward controlling the environment all the time may become a source of stress for the individual.

Depressed and anxious patients tend to display low levels of environmental mastery, but for certain patients the problem may just be the opposite: an excessive sense of mastery that can lead them to trouble. While Ryff's description of environmental mastery is mostly limited to work environment [3], Jahoda's original conception is broader [2] and deserves to be outlined (table 2).

It may be worth pointing out to the patient that environmental mastery can vary according to the situations. One may be quite adequate at work and inadequate in the family, or vice versa. And if you are able to display environmental mastery in one area, there is no reason why you should not be able to achieve it in another. Seneca's concept that psychological well-being is a learning process and writing can promote this process pervades WBT and is continuously shared with the patient.

Table 3. Personal growth

Impaired level	Balanced level	Excessive level
The person has a sense of being stuck; he/she lacks sense of improvement over time; he/she feels bored and uninterested in life	The person has a sense of continued development; he/she sees self as growing and improving; he/she is open to new experiences	The person is unable to elaborate past negative experiences; he/she cultivates illusions that clash with reality; he/she sets unrealistic standards and goals

Personal Growth (table 3)

Ryff [3] splits Jahoda's broad dimension concerned with growth, development, and self-actualization [2] into personal growth and purpose in life. Indeed, in the psychotherapeutic process such distinction is important. Patients often tend to emphasize their distance from expected goals much more than the progress that has been made toward goal achievement. A basic impairment that emerges is the inability to identify the similarities between events and situations that were handled successfully in the past and those that are about to come (transfer of experiences). Impairments in perception of personal growth and environmental mastery thus tend to interact in a dysfunctional way. A university student who is unable to realize the common contents and methodological similarities between the exams he/she successfully passed and the ones that are to be given shows impairments in both environmental mastery and personal growth. The following example provides an illustration of these mechanisms.

The director of a small branch of a bank came to see me. His problem seemed to be paradoxical. Unexpectedly he was going to be promoted to direct a central section of the bank dealing with foreign currencies and financial operations. He went to see the general manager and tried to decline the offer: 'I am very grateful for this opportunity. However, I am in my mid-fifties and I am sure there are better prepared and younger people who could take the position. I am fine where I am.' He added to me: 'I do not know why they picked me: I do not know any foreign language, I have no previous experience with currencies, and I am not good with computers, which is essential in that section.' I also thought that it was quite strange (by the way, this episode which happened many years ago and which was reinforced by many others that occurred subsequently gave me some

Table 4. Goals of session 4

1	Checking how the time period between the sessions went for the patient in general
2	Review of the well-being diary and of the difficulties related to its completion
3	Enhancing the understanding of which feelings and experiences make the patient feel better, including optimal experiences
4	Beginning the cognitive restructuring of the thoughts and/or behaviors that led to a premature interruption of well-being, also by writing on the observer's column
5	Introducing one or two psychological dimensions of well-being according to the material that is presented
6	Continuing with homework assignments (well-being diary, activity encouragement and scheduling, graded task assignments)

insight as to why banks go the way they do). The general manager, however, told him that he could not stay where he was: he could either accept the new position or opt for early retirement (a solution that the patient, whose son and daughter were in college, could not afford). He had always suffered from generalized anxiety, but that situation transformed his anxiety into panic. He had trouble sleeping and also felt that the somatic components of anxiety were overwhelming. In particular, he did not know what to do and feared the potential humiliations that might arise from the new position. We started WBT, but I also gave him the suggestion to accept the new position. 'We will work together and try to cope with the new situation', which we did. After 3 months, my patient was called by the general manager. While he was walking along the long corridor, he thought of that damn psychiatrist who made him accept and be exposed to an impending humiliation. However, the general manager just wanted to congratulate him on how things were going. He could not believe it: 'How is it possible? I have not learned any language, I still understand little of foreign currencies, and I avoid the computer as much as possible.' Going back to his office, he thought of his diary and realized, 'I am very good in my relationships with clients and I know how to create a good team atmosphere, which is exactly what my super-technical predecessor did not have. Other people can take care of the actual work.' Without WBT, this bank employee's unawareness of transfer of experiences and neglect of his skills would have probably resulted in avoidance and in a self-perpetuating sense of inadequacy.

There may also be cases where people set unrealistic standards for their performances, deny negative past experiences, and overestimate their potential ('I am ready to handle anything'). The process of personal growth requires appraisal of both positive and negative experiences, successes, and failures. If it is one-sided (negative or positive), it will lead to recurring mistakes both in professional and sentimental life. Held [6] described the 'tyranny of positive attitudes in United States'. WBT has little to share with 'thinking positive' and much of the positive psychology movement in North America. It does not promote unquestioned optimism and exposure to life's challenges, but attempts to help the individual in his/her everyday struggles.

Graded task assignment may then be pursued. It may involve taking advantage of opportunities, meeting some reasonable challenges, and introducing changes in a very repetitive life. Or it may encompass a decrease in work or family involvement, refraining from excessive and/or untimely challenges, and finding some room for rest and leisure.

The patient is asked to continue the diary, paying particular attention to the psychological dimensions of well-being that have been discussed, and to come back in 2 weeks.

The main goals of the fourth session are summarized in table 4.

References

1 Wright JH, McCray LW: Breaking free from depression. Pathways to wellness. New York, Guilford Press, 2012.
2 Jahoda M: Current Concepts of Positive Mental Health. New York, Basic Books, 1958.
3 Ryff CD: Psychological well-being revisited: advances in the science and practice of eudaimonia. Psychother Psychosom 2014;83:10–28.
4 Fava GA, Tomba E: Increasing psychological well-being and resilience by psychotherapeutic methods. J Pers 2009;77:1903–1934.
5 Ruini C, Fava GA: The individualized and cross-cultural roots of Well-Being Therapy; in Fava GA, Ruini C (eds): Increasing Psychological Well-Being in Clinical and Educational Settings. Dordrecht, Springer, 2014, pp 21–39.
6 Held BS: The tyranny of positive attitudes in America. J Clin Psychol 2002;58:965–992.

Chapter 9
Session 5

During this session the clinician reviews the patient's efforts to monitor interruption of his/her well-being. Techniques to avoid these interruptions are reviewed and reinforced. The therapist and the patient focus on the key areas of psychological well-being (environmental mastery, personal growth, purpose in life, autonomy, self-acceptance, and positive relations with others) that are most relevant to the patient's current issues. In this chapter, I will discuss purpose in life and autonomy, but, as I stated before, in no way does this reflect a prearranged order. Dimensions of psychological well-being should be introduced only if and when they can be found in the material brought in by the patient.

As in the previous sessions, the clinician first asks how the past 2 weeks went and if any difficulty was encountered in completing the homework. At this point in treatment, the patient is expected to be able to readily identify instances of well-being, to be aware of what leads to their interruptions (thoughts and/or behaviors), and to implement alternative strategies (observer's column). Such strategies are generally applied retrospectively (when the patient reflects on past events), but, in due course, the patient may be able to implement them at the time automatic thoughts and/or avoidance behaviors actually occur. As an athlete first learns how to perform certain actions in training and then applies these in the actual game, the patient learns to implement the new insights into practice.

Table 1. Purpose in life

Impaired level	Balanced level	Excessive level
The person lacks a sense of meaning in life; he/she has few goals or aims, and lacks sense of direction	The person has goals in life and feels there is meaning to their present and past life	The person has unrealistic expectations and hopes; he/she is constantly dissatisfied with performance and is unable to recognize failures

The therapist reviews the patient's entries in the well-being diary and helps the patient to make optimal use of cognitive behavior therapy (CBT) techniques to counteract automatic thoughts and avoidance behaviors. This is achieved by discussion and interaction, as well as by writing the most important points in the diary. If the patient is geared towards completing the observer's column, only a brief review of examples from the patient's diary is necessary. However, if the patient seems to be struggling with one or more phases of the process, the therapist should then make wide use of examples and metaphors to achieve this goal.

Strategies (used in sessions and at home) to move the patient toward optimal functioning in well-being are discussed. In addition to environmental mastery and personal growth, which I discussed in the previous chapter, purpose in life and autonomy [1–4] are described here.

Purpose in Life (table 1)

An underlying assumption of psychological therapies (whether pharmacological or psychotherapeutic) is to restore premorbid functioning. In case of treatments which emphasize self-help, such as cognitive behavioral, therapy itself offers a sense of direction and hence a short-term goal. However, this may not persist when acute symptoms abate and/or premorbid functioning is suboptimal. Patients may perceive a lack of sense of direction and may devalue their function in life [3]. This occurs particularly when levels of environmental mastery, personal growth, and purpose in life are impaired (fig. 1). Here we start to realize that psychological dimensions of well-being interact with each other and that this interaction produces clinical effects.

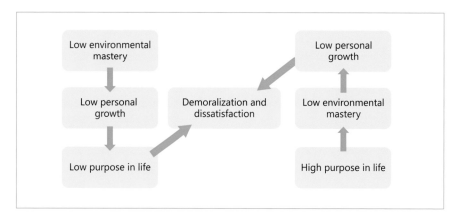

Fig. 1. Pathways to demoralization and dissatisfaction.

Levels of purpose in life may also be unrealistically high and hopes may be excessive. Individuals with a strong determination in realizing one (or more) life goal(s) could become completely engaged in these activities with persistence and abnegation even in the face of major obstacles [4]. While such persistence may foster important professional achievements, it may also lead to neglect of other areas, such as interpersonal relationships and leisure time. 'I'll be the best' may be a good initial stimulus, but sooner or later a person should come to a more realistic appraisal ('I may not be the best, but I do a decent job'). The sobering effects of difficulties and failures are hindered by denial. As depicted figure 1, demoralization and dissatisfaction may then ensue. For example, when high levels of purpose in life are strongly associated with professional goals, retirement may be a very difficult transition to go through. The goal of the therapist is thus to broaden the domains of purpose in life.

Autonomy (table 2)

It is a frequent clinical observation that patients may exhibit a pattern whereby a perceived lack of self-worth leads to unassertive behavior. For instance, patients may hide their opinions or preferences, go along with a situation that is not in their best interests, or consistently put their needs behind the needs of others. This pattern undermines environmental mastery and purpose in life,

Table 2. Autonomy

Impaired level	Balanced level	Excessive level
The person is overconcerned with the expectations and evaluations of others; he/she relies on the judgment of others to make important decisions	The person is independent; he/she is able to resist social pressures; regulates behavior and self by personal standards	The person is unable to get along with other people, to work in a team, to learn from others; he/she is unable to ask for advice or help

Table 3. Goals of session 5

1	Checking how the time period between the sessions went for the patient in general
2	Review of the well-being diary and potential difficulties related to its completion
3	Enhancing understanding and pursuing of optimal experiences
4	Continuing cognitive restructuring of the thoughts and behaviors leading to a premature interruption of well-being, also by writing in the observer's column
5	Introducing further dimensions of psychological well-being according to the material that is presented and discussing how these dimensions can be modulated
6	Continuing with homework assignments (well-being diary, activity encouragement and scheduling, graded task assignments)

which in turn may affect autonomy since these dimensions are highly correlated in clinical populations. Such attitudes may not be obvious to patients who hide their considerable need for social approval. A patient who tries to please everyone is likely to fail to achieve this goal, and the unavoidable conflicts that may ensue can result in chronic dissatisfaction and frustration. Individuals with impaired levels of autonomy are likely to be exploited at work and to get burdened by excessive loads.

On the other hand, individuals may develop the conviction that they should rely only on themselves for solving problems and difficulties, and are thus unable to ask for advice or help. They carry unbearable loads (e.g., as caregivers of one or both parents with invalidating medical illnesses) and wonder why they feel exhausted. Individuals with excessive levels of autonomy are unable to get along with other people, work in teams, or maintain intimate relationships because they are constantly fighting for their opinions and independence [4].

In the course of therapy the patient is confronted with the fact that his/her cognitive schemas and beliefs, as well as behaviors related to psychological well-being, may not be optimal. Like automatic thoughts that derive their destructive strength from the fact of being unchallenged by the individual, the patient is often unaware and has never been challenged on his/her personal constructs of well-being. The CBT techniques that I have described in the previous chapter are very helpful in cognitive restructuring, activity scheduling, and graded task assignments. The concept of 'self-therapy' is adequately reinforced. Graded task assignments may involve learning to resist social pressures ('I must do it because my friend expects me to do it and she will think I let her down otherwise'), with the resulting involvement in activities that are too stressful or unpleasant. Or they may involve asking for help or advice, or setting more realistic goals.

The patient is asked to continue the diary, paying particular attention to the psychological dimensions of well-being that have been discussed, and to come back in 2 weeks.

The main goals of the fifth session are summarized in table 3.

References

1 Jahoda M: Current Concepts of Positive Mental Health. New York, Basic Books, 1958.
2 Ryff CD: Psychological well-being revisited: advances in the science and practice of eudaimonia. Psychother Psychosom 2014;83:10–28.
3 Fava GA, Tomba E: Increasing psychological well-being and resilience by psychotherapeutic methods. J Pers 2009;77:1903–1934.
4 Ruini C, Fava GA: The individualized and cross-cultural roots of Well-Being Therapy; in Fava GA, Ruini C (eds): Increasing Psychological Well-Being in Clinical and Educational Settings. Dordrecht, Springer, 2014, pp 21–39.

Chapter 10

Session 6

During this session the clinician continues to review the patient's efforts to contrast interruptions of well-being and to apply this contrast to live situations, and not only retrospectively. The patient is also encouraged to accept challenges that appear to be in line with his/her abilities and to get exposed to situations that are unnecessarily avoided. The therapist and the patient focus on the key areas of psychological well-being that are the most relevant to the patient's current issues. In this chapter, I will complete their description by outlining self-acceptance and positive relations with others. As already emphasized, in no way does this reflect a prearranged order to be followed in the sessions. The areas are discussed only in relation to the material brought in by the patient.

As in the previous sessions, the clinician first asks about the preceding 2 weeks and whether any difficulties or doubts were encountered in completing the homework. At this point in treatment the patient is expected to be able to readily identify instances of well-being and optimal experiences, be aware of what leads to their interruptions (thoughts and/or behaviors), develop alternative ways of thinking (observer's interpretation of the situation), and implement behaviors that may increase the likelihood of well-being and optimal experiences. The therapist reviews the patient's entries in the well-being diary and helps the patient make optimal use of cognitive behavior therapy techniques to counteract automatic thoughts and avoidance behaviors.

Strategies (used in sessions and at home) to move the patient toward optimal functioning in well-being are discussed in this chapter, with particular reference to self-acceptance and positive relations with others [1–4].

Table 1. Self-acceptance

Impaired level	Balanced level	Excessive level
The person feels dissatisfied with himself/herself; he/she is disappointed with what has occurred in his/her past life; he/she wishes to be different	The person accepts his/her good and bad qualities and feels positive about his/her past life	The person has difficulties in admitting own mistakes; he/she attributes all problems to others' faults

Self-Acceptance (table 1)

Patients may maintain unrealistically high standards and expectations, driven by perfectionistic attitudes (which reflect lack of self-acceptance) and/or endorsement of external instead of personal standards (which reflect lack of autonomy). As a result, any instance of well-being is neutralized by a chronic dissatisfaction with oneself. A person may set unrealistic standards for his/her performance. For instance, it is a frequent clinical observation that patients with social phobia tend to aspire to outstanding social performance (being sharp, humorous, etc.) and are not satisfied with average performances (despite the fact that these latter would not put them under the spotlights, which could be seen as their apparent goal). The opposite situation may ensue when an apparently inflated self-esteem (as in cyclothymia and bipolar disorder) may clash with reality. The person's inability to admit his/her own mistakes makes him/her attribute all problems to others' faults and deficiencies. So, for instance, repeated inability to get a permanent position at work is always due to envious colleagues who put the person under a bad light and not to counterproductive behavior.

Positive Relations with Others (table 2)

Interpersonal relationships may be influenced by strongly held attitudes of which the patient may be unaware and which may be dysfunctional, as the following example illustrates.

> Ann is a young clerk who recently got married after a series of unsuccessful relationships. She is convinced she has found the right man and wants her marriage to be perfect. One of the pillars of perfection would be to be open to each other about how they

Table 2. Positive relations with others

Impaired level	Balanced level	Excessive level
The person has few close, trusting relationships with others; he/she finds it difficult to be open	The person has trusting relationships with others; he/she is concerned about the welfare of others; he/she understands the give and take of human relationships	The person sacrifices his/her needs and well-being for those of others; low self-esteem and sense of worthlessness induce excessive readiness to forgive

feel. She and her husband would always share how they feel. Yet this seems to be putting their relationship under considerable strain. Ann's husband seems to be hurt by some of her comments and remarks, and reacts by staying silent. Ann concludes that once again she has failed and that she is simply unable to build a solid link with a man.

The example illustrates how a person may set unrealistic standards (perfect wife and perfect marriage) and, driven by a perfectionistic attitude, may be looking for trouble. At the remark of the therapist that voicing anything that comes to mind is not a great strategy since the majority of our thoughts are meaningless emotional expressions that need to be adjusted in due course (internal dialogue), the patient is very surprised. She relies on the total suppression of her bad qualities that should have magically disappeared after the wedding and has no cognitive instruments for correcting and/or balancing her thoughts. At the same time, she may avoid pursuing social plans which involve other people and may lack sources of comparison. Impairments in self-acceptance (with the resulting belief of being rejectable and unlovable) may further undermine positive relations with others. There is a large body of literature [5] on the buffering effects of social integration, social network properties, and perceived support. Family relationships and family life have also been extensively studied for their health consequences, even though the focus has been on the negative (e.g., divorce, separation) and how they compromise health [6], with much less attention given to the ways in which family life contributes to human flourishing [7]. Improvements in family functioning may facilitate the recovery process in depression [8].

On the other hand, excessive levels of empathy, altruism, and generosity, which are usually considered to be positive, may be detrimental. For instance, patients may report a sense of guilt for not being able to help someone (who could hardly be helped in that specific situation) or to forgive an offence. An in-

Table 3. Goals of session 6

1	Checking the general status of the patient
2	Review of the well-being diary and pursuit of optimal experiences
3	Review of cognitive restructuring and in vivo contrast of automatic thoughts
4	Introducing and/or improving dysfunctional dimensions of psychological well-being according to the material that is presented
5	Continuing with homework assignments (well-being diary, activity encouragement and scheduling, graded task assignments)

dividual with a strong prosocial attitude can sacrifice his/her needs and well-being for those of others and become overconcerned and overwhelmed by others' problems and distress. Finally, a generalized tendency to forgive others and be grateful to benefactors could mask low self-esteem and a low sense of personal worth [4].

The patient is thus confronted with alternative constructs and behaviors. He/she is asked to continue the diary, paying particular attention to the dimensions of well-being that have been discussed in the session. The concept of self-therapy is reinforced. Graded task assignments may involve pursuing social opportunities (e.g., making phone calls to friends they had neglected) or limiting excessive sacrifices. If appropriate, the patient may also be asked to come back in 3–4 weeks instead of using the customary 2-week interval.

The main goals of the sixth session are summarized in table 3.

References

1 Jahoda M: Current Concepts of Positive Mental Health. New York, Basic Books, 1958.
2 Ryff CD: Psychological well-being revisited: advances in the science and practice of eudaimonia. Psychother Psychosom 2014;83:10–28.
3 Fava GA, Tomba E: Increasing psychological well-being and resilience by psychotherapeutic methods. J Pers 2009;77:1903–1934
4 Ruini C, Fava GA: The individualized and cross-cultural roots of Well-Being Therapy; in Fava GA, Ruini C (eds): Increasing Psychological Well-Being in Clinical and Educational Settings. Dordrecht, Springer, 2014, pp 21–39.
5 Uchino BN, Cacioppo JT, Kiecolt-Glaser JK: The relationship between social support and physiological processes: a review with emphasis on underlying mechanisms and implications for health. Psychol Bull 1996;119:488–531.
6 Fava GA, Sonino N: Psychosomatic medicine. Int J Clin Practice 2010;64:999–1001.
7 Ryff CD, Singer BH: Interpersonal flourishing: a positive health agenda for the new millennium. Pers Soc Psychol Rev 2000;4:30–44.
8 Fabbri S, Fava GA, Rafanelli C, Tomba E: Family intervention approach to loss of clinical effect during long-term antidepressant treatment: a pilot study. J Clin Psychiatry 2007;68:1348–1351.

Chapter 11
Session 7

During this session the clinician reviews the patient's progress. The patient is expected to rate progress that has been made and to identify areas that still require work and adjustments. The therapist reminds the patient that sustained feelings of well-being should still be the exception instead of the rule, and that progress is likely to take an up-and-down course. What really matters are the new insights that may ensue, which only continuous training (self-therapy) may sustain and make lasting. One should not become a radically different person to experience well-being. On the contrary: it is the removal of cognitive and behavioral obstacles that may unravel and free the person you are. Patients may attribute much or all of their progress to the therapist's efforts and/or expertise. In such cases it is critical to reinforce with the patient that he/she has done the majority of work outside the sessions. The therapist can review the initial part of the diary, gains achieved, and techniques used by the patient to make this progress. Particular emphasis is placed on highlighting successful use of alternative strategies in everyday life. The patient has learned a lot and is getting ready to continue self-therapy on his/her own.

The clinician and the patient focus on the areas of psychological well-being (environmental mastery, personal growth, purpose in life, autonomy, self-acceptance, and positive relations with others) that have been discussed in relation to the well-being diary. At this stage it is generally possible to have a profile of the dimensions of psychological well-being for the specific individual, not only as to their impaired or excessive levels, but also as to their variable interactions. This means that you may find a person with excessive levels in some dimensions, impairments in other aspects, and unaffected areas. For instance, an individual with rigidity and incapacity to admit mistakes (excessive levels of self-acceptance), and apparently adequate environmental mastery, is likely to be frustrated in interpersonal relationships, pursuit of goals, and personal growth. The work with Well-Being Therapy (WBT) may disclose that the environmental mastery is more apparent than real, and low self-esteem and worthlessness are undermining the psychological balance.

Excessively elevated levels of positive emotions can become detrimental and are more connected with mental disorders and impaired functioning, as Wood and Tarrier [1] described. In 1991, Garamoni et al. [2] suggested that healthy functioning is characterized by an optimal balance of positive and negative cognitions or affects, and that psychopathology is marked by deviations from the optimal balance. Marie Jahoda [3] outlined a central synthesizing psychological dimension of well-being, which she called 'integration', with emphasis on the changeable balance of psychic forces (flexibility), a unifying outlook on life which guides actions and feelings for shaping future accordingly, and resistance to stress (resilience and tolerance for anxiety or frustration). It is not simply a generic (and useless) invitation to avoiding excesses and extremes. It is how the individual adjusts the psychological dimensions of well-being to changing needs.

Jahoda was born in Vienna in 1907 and grew up there being both Jewish and a socialist. She was imprisoned by the Austro-fascist regime, but was able to escape to England in 1937. After World War II she became Professor of Social Psychology at Columbia University in New York. She went back to England in the 1960s and started a political career. Her life is by itself an indication of the flexibility and change in focus that the pursuit of psychological well-being entails. As a result, it is not sufficient to detect impaired or excessive levels of the dimensions of psychological well-being. It is also important to appraise how they interact and develop in changing situations, which is subsumed by Jahoda's concept of integration [3].

In our first pilot study on WBT that was published in 1998 [4], I gained some important insights. First, psychological well-being, as measured by the Psychological Well-Being Scales (PWB) [5], could be increased by a short course of WBT (one might have thought that we were dealing with stable traits that were not amenable to modification). Second, standard cognitive behavior therapy

(CBT) focused on distress could also achieve such a result, even though not to the same significant degree as WBT. Finally, the various psychological dimensions encompassed by Ryff's PWB [5] appeared to be strongly related among themselves and to both observer and self-rated measures of distress [6].

At this point in time, I like to share with my patients these insights, highlighting three key messages:

1 One can learn to feel better (Seneca's concept of well-being as a training process), but needs to work on it with homework.
2 Any small improvement in one area can result in amelioration of other areas not subject to specific work.
3 Different strategies, whether cognitive or behavioral, may yield similar results. Therefore, it is important to extend efforts to many areas with different methods.

As to this last issue, it is not surprising that WBT has similarities with other approaches that have been developed in the psychotherapeutic field.

An approach that was developed before WBT, interpersonal psychotherapy [7], has its focus on improving social adjustment. It may overlap with WBT work on positive relations with others, even though interpersonal psychotherapy does not include specific homework. Interpersonal functioning, however, is only one of the working areas of WBT. WBT in turn would not be suitable for coping with recent losses (an early emphasis on well-being could be counterproductive).

There are also overlaps with other techniques that have been recently reviewed by MacLeod and Luzon [8] as to their implication for well-being:

1 Behavioral activation [9] assumes that people may avoid situations that could potentially give them pleasure or a sense of achievement.
2 Mindfulness-based cognitive therapy [10] is built on the Buddhist philosophy of a good life; however, it has some elements of well-being that are not specifically addressed. Its specificity (superiority to active control groups) has been recently challenged [11].
3 Acceptance and commitment therapy (ACT) is the integration of behavioral theories of change with mindfulness and acceptance strategies, with the goal of improving flexibility [12]. There is some overlap with WBT self-acceptance. However, ACT argues that attempts at changing thoughts can be counterproductive and instead it encourages awareness and acceptance through mindfulness practice. Therefore, the approach is almost opposite to WBT. Also the specificity of ACT compared to CBT has been challenged [13].

Table 1. Goals of session 7

1	Checking the general status of the patient and feelings about ending therapy soon
2	Review of the well-being diary and pursuit of optimal experiences
3	Review of cognitive restructuring and in vivo contrast of automatic thoughts
4	Reinforcing strategies for improving psychological well-being
5	Continuing with homework assignments (well-being diary, exposure, activity scheduling)
6	Reinforcing willingness to keep on working (self-therapy) after therapy has ended

There are also other psychotherapeutic approaches, such as Padesky and Mooney's Strengths-Based CBT [14], that have been proposed to increase well-being, but that await adequate validation. Their role in clinical practice is still to be determined.

However, even though techniques may overlap, the focus of WBT (self-observation of psychological well-being) is completely different from the other, distress-oriented approaches. What distinguishes WBT, particularly in the final sessions, is its integrated focus which is not limited to only one aspect (e.g., self-acceptance), based on Jahoda's comprehensive framework [3]. Its focus is individualized and depends on the specific profile of the patient. The CBT techniques that are selected are finalized to this purpose.

At the end of the session, the patient is praised for the work done, is asked to continue the diary and to come back in a month.

The main goals of the seventh session are summarized in table 1.

References

1 Wood AM, Tarrier N: Positive clinical psychology. Clin Psychol Rev 2010;30:819–829.
2 Garamoni GL, Reynolds CF 3rd, Thase ME, Frank E, Berman SR, Fasiczka AL: The balance of positive and negative affects in major depression: a further test of the States of Mind model. Psychiatry Res 1991;39:99–108.
3 Jahoda M: Current Concepts of Positive Mental Health. New York, Basic Books, 1958.
4 Fava GA, Rafanelli C, Cazzaro M, Conti S, Grandi S: Well-Being Therapy. A novel psychotherapeutic approach for residual symptoms of affective disorders. Psychol Med 1998;28:475–480.
5 Ryff CD: Psychological well-being revisited: advances in the science and practice of eudaimonia. Psychother Psychosom 2014;83:10–28.
6 Rafanelli C, Park SK, Ruini C, Ottolini F, Cazzaro M, Fava GA: Rating well-being and distress. Stress Med 2000;16:55–61.

7   Klerman GL, Weissman MM, Rounsaville BJ, Chevron ES: Interpersonal Psychotherapy of Depression. New York, Basic Books, 1984.

8   MacLeod AK, Luzon O: The place of psychological well-being in cognitive therapy; in Fava GA, Ruini C (eds): Increasing Psychological Well-Being in Clinical and Educational Settings. Dordrecht, Springer, 2014, pp 41–55.

9   Jacobson NS, Martell CR, Dimidjian S: Behavioral activation treatment for depression. Clin Psychol Soc Pract 2001;8:225–270.

10 Segal ZV, Williams JMG, Teasdale JD: Mindfulness-Based Cognitive Therapy for Depression. New York, Guilford Press, 2002.

11 Goyal M, Singh S, Sibinga EMS, Gould NF, Rowland-Seymour A, Sharma R, Berger Z, Sleicher D, Maron DD, Shihab HM, Ranasinghe PD, Linn S, Saha S, Bass EB, Haythornthwaite JA: Meditation programs for psychological stress and well-being: a systematic review and meta-analysis. JAMA Intern Med 2014;174:357–368.

12 Hayes SC, Strosahal K, Wilson KG: Acceptance and Commitment Therapy. New York, Guilford Press, 1999.

13 Powers MB, Zum Vörde Sive Vörding MB, Emmelkamp PMG: Acceptance and commitment therapy: a meta-analytic review. Psychother Psychosom 2009;78:73–80.

14 Padesky CA, Mooney K: Strengths-based cognitive-behavioural therapy: a four-step model to build resilience. Clin Psychol Psychother 2012;19:283–290.

Chapter 12

Session 8

This represents the last session of this course of psychotherapy. As such it is important to review the clinical situation of the patient and to provide links to the disturbances that brought him/her to seek attention. It is not simply a matter of reviewing what has been learned in therapy and the specific tools that have been acquired, but also the ideal moment for discussing how the therapy may have affected the clinical state of the patient.

Many individuals can only provide a global description of their progress ('I'm feeling better' or 'I can cope better now'). In this case the clinician needs to ask the patient for examples supporting such general statements. This may be performed by going through the well-being diary. The therapist may also write specific statements in the diary, which the patient is likely to check from time to time. Such statements may concern issues such as the reduction of stress that has occurred, a decrease in anxiety and tension, the capability to react to moments of distress, and an improved quality of life. If specific assessment instruments have been used, such as the Clinical Interview for Depression (CID) [1], Psychological Well-Being Scales (PWB) [2], and Symptom Questionnaire (SQ) [3], it may be useful to administer them again and to check the differences with the patient. The 'well-being check' that was described in Chapter 5 may be another helpful comparison to see whether the patient has improved the scores from the first time he/she did it. All these instruments may reinforce a sense of progress associated with Well-Being Therapy (WBT). This is also the time when links to psychotropic medications the patient may be using can be discussed. Such links will be described in Part III of this book, which is concerned with specific clinical disturbances. If the medication has been tapered and/or discontinued, the value of self-therapy is once again underscored:

> As a patient with high blood pressure and/or high cholesterol may have the medication reduced or discontinued by the physician if he/she has been able to lose weight, eat better, and engage in more physical activity, your efforts toward a better psychological functioning have decreased or eliminated the need for medication.

If the condition of the patient has substantially improved, fear of relapse becomes an important source of concern. The fear may be increased by the ending of the therapy, which also provides a reassuring monitoring of the patient's condition (see the initial phase of each session). I do not deny the reality of relapse with generic optimism ('everything will be OK'). The therapist can tell the patient:

> Relapse may occur, but we have decreased its likelihood. Things do not necessarily work out at the first attempt. If relapse occurs, we may provide a timely treatment and see together what did not work and why. We always have at least a second chance.

Another issue that is important to outline is the flexibility in terms of number of sessions. There are patients who need fewer than 8 sessions and others who require a more extended treatment (12 or more sessions). I also make clear that 'booster' therapy sessions are always available:

> This is our last scheduled session. It means that this is the last session that has been planned. But this does not mean that it is our last session. If we schedule an appointment in 2 months, for instance, maybe nothing important happens. And 2 weeks later there is something you would like to discuss with me. So the best thing to do is call me whenever you need me and we can see each other again. In any event I would like to see you in a year to see how much you have progressed with self-therapy.

At times, in my practice, patients call me up, and often only a brief telephone exchange is necessary. Other times we see each other again for a rehearsal of the well-being strategies while coping with a difficult situation. There are also instances when the patient wants to see me for sharing some very positive events that happened to them (and this is a very rewarding occurrence). Finally, there are patients whom I do not see or hear from before the 1-year follow-up assessment, which I always like to perform, with an additional 2 year follow-up visit if possible.

Table 1. Kellner's scale for change after treatment (modified from [4])

A lot worse		Worse		Same		Better		A lot better
9	8	7	6	5	4	3	2	1

So far I have considered the situation where WBT has yielded an improvement in the patient's sense of well-being and clinical condition. Such improvement may be deemed to be satisfactory by the clinician and the patient. As I explained in Chapter 4, even a good degree of response, however, may not be sufficient, particularly in chronic and complex conditions, and other lines of therapy may be planned and discussed with the patient. However, we must also consider the possibility that the patient has not displayed any improvement or had a worsening in his/her clinical situations. Robert Kellner devised a very simple observer-rated scale for rating change after treatment (table 1) [4].

Any type of treatment is unlikely to benefit more than two thirds of the patients (see Chapter 4), and there is no exception with WBT. Dropout is a substantial problem with any type of psychotherapy and this was found to occur also with WBT in controlled trials, even though not to a degree that was significantly higher than a control condition. Another potential source of failure is the lack of compliance with the homework that is a part of WBT (e.g. the patient may not work with the diary in a sufficient way). But even when compliance is good, the patient (and the clinician) may be disappointed:

> I was really believing in this new approach after all the different types of drug treatment that I received and the courses of psychotherapy that I underwent. But I see that nothing has changed and that my situation is hopeless.

Not surprisingly the failure of expectations can lead to a worsening of the clinical situation. It is also possible that the therapy triggered some negative reactions in the patient (as in the case described in Chapter 2). In all these cases it is important to share with the patient that no treatment is universally effective and that something might have gone wrong with this treatment. However, other therapists and approaches may succeed where one fails. Referral to an independent clinician for evaluation may be something to be considered as well.

Marie Jahoda [5] observed that psychological treatment of mental patients is guided by the search for a conceptual formulation that acts as a 'unifying principle in terms of which the apparently most bizarrely inconsistent manifesta-

Table 2. Goals of session 8

1	Checking the patient's feeling about ending the therapy
2	Review of the well-being diary
3	Pointing to improvements that have occurred in the various areas of well-being and in the amount of distress
4	Discussing difficulties that limited the self-therapy with WBT
5	Emphasizing the importance to keep on working (self-therapy) afterwards
6	Confirming availability for future 'booster' sessions, if and when needed; arranging for follow-up
7	Placing the experience of WBT in the treatment history of the patient, including potential prospects of other lines of treatment

tions of personality can be understood to hang together' [5, p. 36]. Psychotherapeutic schools often purport to possess such a unifying outlook and to entail universal solution to patients' problems. WBT, by monitoring well-being instead of distress, may offer a helpful framework for some patients, may yield little improvement in other individuals, and may even be harmful in other situations.

Going back, however, to the favorable and positive outcome, at the end of the session the patient is praised for the work done and reminded that the therapist is available for future 'booster' sessions.

The main goals of the eighth session are summarized in table 2.

References

1 Guidi J, Fava GA, Bech P, Paykel ES: The Clinical Interview for Depression: a comprehensive review of studies and clinimetric properties. Psychother Psychosom 2011;80:10–27.

2 Ryff CD: Psychological well-being revisited: advances in the science and practice of eudaimonia. Psychother Psychosom 2014;83:10–28.

3 Kellner R: A symptom questionnaire. J Clin Psychiatry 1987;48:268–274.

4 Kellner R: Improvement criteria in drug trials with neurotic patients. Part 2. Psychol Med 1972;2:73–80.

5 Jahoda M: Current Concepts of Positive Mental Health. New York, Basic Books, 1958.

Chapter 13
The Four-Session Program

In many of the clinical controlled studies that have been performed, the application of Well-Being Therapy (WBT) occurred after a course of cognitive behavior therapy (CBT) (see Chapter 3). The basic principle that guided this strategy was to address distress first by psychological methods as the most urgent priority and impairments in well-being at a later point in time. In these cases, when WBT comes into the picture the patient is already familiar with self-observation (the diary), the monitoring of automatic thoughts, and the various strategies for counteracting automatic thoughts (observer's column).

The therapist then uses an introduction such as follows:

> So far you have learned and practiced techniques to help you feel better during times of distress. We have focused on your problems and difficulties. Now it is time to change our target. We will concentrate on your well-being and how to increase it.

Modifications of this introduction can be made as necessary, but the essential message should remain: we are switching gears. The sequence of the sessions is as follows.

First Session

The clinician checks the general status of the patient and his/her level of mastery of the CBT techniques. It is important to be sure that no major difficulties are encountered in completing the homework. If the therapist has the perception that the patient's mastery of CBT is still incomplete, it is better to postpone the switch to WBT. It is far more productive spending 2–4 additional sessions than embarking on a new strategy with insufficient preparation.

Table 1. Goals of session 1

1	Checking the general status of the patient
2	Checking the patient's mastery in understanding and applying CBT strategies
3	Introducing the change in focus of therapy (well-being instead of distress)
4	Providing information about the structure and modalities of WBT, including estimated number of sessions and expected homework
5	Giving homework assignments (well-being diary), including monitoring of instances of well-being, thoughts and/or behaviors leading to their premature interruption, and the observer's column

If the patient shows a satisfactory mastery of the CBT strategies, the clinician may go on with switching to WBT, with an introduction similar to the one that was previously described. The patient is asked to use the same diary he worked with before. However, he/she is asked to record circumstances of well-being and the automatic thoughts that led to their premature interruption, and attempt an observer's interpretation of the situation. The assignments of sessions 1 (Chapter 5), 2 (Chapter 6), 3 (Chapter 7), and 4 (Chapter 8) are thus provided from the very beginning in this initial session. The patient is asked to work on the diary, as he/she did in the first part of the therapy, and to come back in 2 weeks.

The main goals of the first session are summarized in table 1.

Second Session

The session is focused on making the patient aware of having episodes of well-being and on understanding what leads to their premature interruption. The patient should realize that automatic thoughts not only trigger distress, but may spoil positive moments in one's life.

The patient presents the data collected in his/her diary, which is now defined as a well-being diary. Examination of entries may lead to introducing the concept of optimal experiences and how these should be pursued. Further, the role of avoidance behavior is underscored. If the material that is brought by the patient is appropriate, one or at most two of the psychological dimensions developed by Jahoda [1] and elaborated by Ryff [2] are introduced. The therapist plays an active

Table 2. Goals of session 2

1	Checking the general status of the patient
2	Review of the well-being diary with particular reference to automatic thoughts, avoidance behavior, and the observer's interpretation
3	Introducing the concept of optimal experience
4	Introducing one or two psychological dimensions of well-being according to the material that is presented
5	Continuing with homework assignments (well-being diary, activity encouragement and scheduling)

Table 3. Goals of session 3

1	Checking the general status of the patient, with particular reference to improvements in the duration of well-being episodes
2	Review of the well-being diary with particular reference to automatic thoughts, avoidance behavior, and the observer's interpretation
3	Encouraging pursuit of optimal experiences
4	Review of cognitive restructuring, reinforcing behavioral strategies for improving well-being
5	Modulating dimensions of psychological well-being according to the material that is presented
6	Continuing with homework assignments (well-being diary, exposure, activity scheduling)
7	Checking the patient's feelings about ending therapy soon

part in writing comments in the patient's diary. The patient is praised for the work that was done, and is asked to continue the diary and to come back in 2 weeks.

The goals of the second session are summarized in table 2.

Third Session

In this session the therapist plays a more active role in pointing out alternative cognitive and behavioral strategies to the patient. An example would be a patient receiving praise from a work supervisor with subsequent feelings of well-being, only to be interrupted by the thought 'he gives praise to everybody' or 'he only wants me to stay late tonight'. The clinician shows how CBT techniques can be applied to that situation. There is a further deepening of psychological dimen-

Table 4. Goals of session 4

1	Checking the patient's feeling about ending therapy
2	Review of the well-being diary, underscoring improvements that have occurred in the various areas of well-being and in the amount of distress
3	Discussing difficulties that limited self-therapy with WBT
4	Modulating psychological dimensions of well-being by cognitive restructuring
5	Confirming availability for future 'booster' sessions; arranging for follow-up

sions of well-being, always according to the material that is presented and not in a prearranged way (see Chapters 5–7). The clinician helps the patient in modulating these dimensions, avoiding polarities of levels that are too high or too low, or that are simply not suitable for the life situation.

The patient is praised for the work done, and is asked to continue his/her homework and to come back in 2 weeks.

The goals of the third session are summarized in table 3.

Fourth Session

This represents the last session of a course of psychotherapy that involved CBT in the first 4–8 sessions. As described in Chapter 12, it is important to review the clinical situation of the patient and the progress that has been made.

The value of continuing self-therapy after the session is underscored. As was the case for the duration of CBT, it is important to be flexible as to the duration of treatment (some patients may require a longer course of WBT). It is important to also make clear that 'booster' therapy sessions are always available (see Chapter 12). The therapist reviews the diary entries and provides further alternatives in terms of cognition and behavior to those reported by the patients. Modulation of psychological dimensions that are raised by the patient's material is also performed.

The main goals of the fourth session are summarized in table 4.

References

1 Jahoda M: Current Concepts of Positive Mental Health. New York, Basic Books, 1958.
2 Ryff CD: Psychological well-being revisited: advances in the science and practice of eudaimonia. Psychother Psychosom 2014;83:10–28.

Chapter 14
Depression

Major depressive disorder is a highly prevalent condition in the general population. Approximately 8 of 10 people experiencing a depressive illness will have 1 or more episodes during their lifetime, i.e., a recurrent major depressive disorder [1]. In some patients, the episodes are separated by many symptom-free years of normal functioning. For others, the episodes become increasingly frequent. The latter course appears to be the more prevalent, both in psychiatric and primary care settings [1, 2].

Partial remission between episodes, not full recovery, appears to be the rule and is associated with residual disability [2]. At least 1 patient out of 3 is likely to relapse within a year [1, 2]. Two major risk factors associated with relapse appear to be the persistence of subthreshold or subclinical symptoms and number of episodes of major depression [2]. As a result, for most people, depression is a lifelong chronic disorder with multiple recurrences [1].

Antidepressant drugs have been advocated as the cure for depression and the best way to prevent relapse. However, antidepressant drugs are more effective than placebo only when depression reaches a certain level of severity (a major depressive disorder) [3], particularly when symptoms such as anorexia, weight loss, middle and late insomnia, and psychomotor disturbances are present [4]. Antidepressant drugs are unlikely to be better than placebo in mild depression [3, 5]; sadness and demoralization are unaffected by their action [4]. If one is sad because he/she was left by a significant other, one may be helped by the idea of taking an antidepressant, but hardly because of a pharmacological action. However, since the early 1990s the availability of antidepressant drugs which were far more tolerable than the traditional ones (the tricyclics) led to their use in mood disturbances that do not reach the severity threshold of major depressive disorders. The duration of antidepressant treatment was also extended to the longest possible time for preventing relapse. Leading journal articles, symposia, and practice guidelines pushed clinicians toward prescribing antidepressant drugs more and more, and for longer and longer.

However, things are not as simple as the propaganda makes them. With long-term treatment, antidepressant drugs may lose efficacy and may induce paradoxical effects and/or resistance [4]. Further, they may work too much: they may induce mania or hypomania or behavioral activation, particularly in younger patients [6], which further complicates the issue.

This is the scenario of the development of the idea of sequential treatment of depression as described in Chapter 1: use of pharmacotherapy in the treatment of an acute episode of depression followed by psychotherapy [including Well-Being Therapy (WBT)] in the residual phase with slow tapering and discontinuation of antidepressant drugs [7]. In this chapter, I will describe the practical application of this approach.

Assessment and Treatment of an Acute Episode

In the past decades, clinical medicine has witnessed the emergence of special interest groups. Corporate interests have fused with academic medicine to create an unhealthy alliance that works against objective reporting of clinical research; sets up meetings and symposia with the specific purpose of selling the participants to the sponsors; gets its prodigal experts into leading roles in journals, medical associations, and nonprofit research organizations; and provides the appropriate degree of rejection of outliers [8]. Massive propaganda has created an automatic thought that is stronger than any attempt at reasoning: each DSM diagnosis should be translated into prescribing action. As a result, when the severity of a major depressive disorder is reached, antidepressant drugs should be prescribed and the physician who does not do it promptly is a criminal. I may be a criminal, but I filter this automatic thought with clinical reasoning.

Table 1. Major depressive disorder: stages of development

1	Prodromal phase
	a. No depressive symptoms (generalized anxiety, irritability, anhedonia, sleep disorders) with mild functional change or decline
	b. Mood symptoms (sad mood, subsyndromal depression)
2.	Major depressive episode
3	Residual phase
	a. No depressive symptoms (sleep disturbance, generalized anxiety, irritability, anorexia, impaired libido)
	b. Mood symptoms (depressed mood, guilt, hopelessness)
	c. Dysthymia
4	a. Recurrent depression
	b. Double depression
5	Chronic major depressive episode (lasting at least 2 years without interruptions)

First of all, it is important to supplement the information provided by an interview leading to DSM diagnoses [9] with a longitudinal view of development of mood disturbances (table 1). Twenty years ago, Robert Kellner and I introduced the concept of staging in psychiatric diagnosis [10], and there is now increasing evidence of its clinical utility [11]. It is important to know where the patient is located in the development of the disorder.

Both pharmacotherapy and certain types of psychotherapy [cognitive behavior therapy (CBT) and interpersonal] are effective in the average case of depression [12]. Antidepressant drugs offer a number of advantages in specific clinical situations:

- They are readily available.
- They can be administered by nonpsychiatric physicians without specialized training.
- They can act in a few weeks.
- The magnitude of benefit of antidepressant medication compared with placebo increases with severity of depressive symptoms [3]; antidepressants are thus the treatment of choice in severe and/or melancholic depression.

There are also disadvantages such as side effects from the drugs and potential interactions with medical conditions. Additionally, if there have been previous unsuccessful trials with medications (table 2), using antidepressant drugs again may cause problems. From a clinical viewpoint it is quite different to use anti-

Table 2. Staging of levels of treatment resistance in unipolar depression

Stage 0	No history of failure to respond to therapeutic trial of antidepressant drugs
Stage 1	Failure of at least one adequate therapeutic trial of antidepressant drugs
Stage 2	Failure of at least two adequate trials of antidepressant drugs
Stage 3	Failure of three or more adequate therapeutic trials of antidepressant drugs
Stage 4	Failure of three or more adequate trials including at least one concerned with augmentation/combination with psychotherapy

depressant drugs in a patient who displayed a positive response to previous therapeutic trials (stage 0) and a patient who failed to respond to various adequate trials (stage 3). In the former case the patient is likely to respond to the same treatment that was effective before, whereas in the latter situation the evidence clearly indicates that the more trials are performed, the more resistant and intolerant to new drug treatments the patient becomes [4].

Evidence-based psychotherapy (particularly CBT and interpersonal therapy) has a few advantages in the treatment of the acute episode [12]:

- It has fewer side effects, particularly in the setting of medical disease.
- It does not seem to induce phenomena of resistance.
- It may yield better long-term prognosis.
  There are also disadvantages [12]:
- Patients need motivation for psychotherapy.
- A competent psychotherapist may not be available.
- Remission from depression tends to be slower than with pharmacotherapy.

Combined treatment (pharmacotherapy and psychotherapy) may offer slight advantages compared to each of the treatments alone in the average case of depression, but it also combines the disadvantages of both approaches.

If depression is severe, I am inclined to prescribe an antidepressant drug. If symptoms are of mild or moderate intensity and appear to be fluctuating, I postpone the prescription and see the patient again after a couple of weeks. If the symptoms have improved to a certain degree, the need for antidepressant drug treatment may be low; in case of persistence (or, at times, worsening) of symptoms, the use of antidepressant drugs appears to be more justified and worth pursuing. The various types of antidepressant drugs may be substantially equivalent in efficacy in the average case of depression [13]. Such an assumption, however, may apply only to the first episode of depression in a patient who has never been treated with antidepressant drugs. Even in this case there are important issues to be considered. Tricyclic antidepressants, despite more side effects, may be more efficacious than second-generation antidepressants in melancholic depression [14].

However, if a patient has already been treated with antidepressant drugs, the choice has to take into account the treatment history of the patient, i.e., whether he/she responded to the drug and/or displayed untoward reactions. Elena Tomba [15] has observed that subjects are generally recruited in a trial irrespective of the treatment history and are thus 'nowhere patients', using an expression that was the title of a Beatles song.

The time of response to antidepressant drugs may be variable, but 3 months appear to be a reasonable time to assess the patient again. This is the time when the sequential strategy begins.

Second-Line Treatment

Before undergoing sequential treatment, patients should have displayed a satisfactory response to antidepressant drug treatment. Therefore, they should have had at least 3 months of drug treatment and no longer be presenting with depressed mood. During pharmacological treatment and clinical management, however, it is essential to introduce the subsequent part of treatment.

A helpful example which was made in an original study [16] was the following:

When I first saw you, you were very depressed. You went off the road. I gave you antidepressant drugs and these put you back on the road. Things are much better now. However, if you keep on driving the way you did, you will go off the road again, sooner or later.

The example outlines the need for lifestyle modification and introduces a sense of control in the patient as to his/her depressive illness. This psychological preparation paves the way for subsequent psychotherapeutic approaches.

Psychotherapeutic intervention extends over 10 sessions, which last between 30 and 45 min each, every other week. The first session is mainly concerned with assessment and introduction of the psychotherapeutic treatment by the therapist, rehearsing the example provided before formal initiation of treatment. Sessions 2–6 are concerned with cognitive behavioral treatment of residual symptoms and lifestyle modification. The last four sessions involve WBT; however, this format is liable to wide variations in relation to the specific characteristics and treatment history of a patient.

Table 3. Example of the assessment diary

Situation	Distress (0–100)	Thoughts
I am watching TV, when the telephone rings	40	Something has certainly happened to…

Session 1

It is of considerable importance to reassess the remitted patient as if he/she were a new patient. This means to go through symptoms in the most recent weeks in a careful way. Exploration should not concern only symptoms which characterize the diagnosis of major depressive disorder, but also those which characterize anxiety disturbances (including phobic and obsessive-compulsive symptoms) and irritability. In the original studies [16, 17] a modified version of Paykel's Clinical Interview for Depression [18] was employed, but other semistructured interviews may be used as long as they are sufficiently comprehensive as to anxiety and irritability. This is the first step in recognizing residual symptomatology, which we expect to find in 80–90% of patients who respond to antidepressant drugs.

The second step deals with self-observation of the patient. He/she is instructed to report in a diary (table 3) all episodes of distress that occur in the following 2 weeks. It is important to emphasize that distress (which is left unspecified) does not need to be prolonged, but may also be short lived. Patients are also instructed to build a list of situations which elicit distress and/or tend to induce avoidance. Each situation should be rated on a scale of 0–100 (0 = no problem; 100 = panic, unbearable distress). Patients are instructed to bring the diary at the next visit.

Let us consider the case of Mike. He is a 44-year-old man who works as a county clerk and has a major depressive disorder of recent onset. He had two previous episodes 1 and 3 years earlier that were treated by his primary care physician with fluvoxamine (100 mg/day) for 4 months each time. Although in this case his physician prescribed fluvoxamine again, he wonders whether a different treatment (perhaps psychotherapy) may be justified. Careful assessment discloses only partial remission after each episode. I confirmed the prescription of fluvoxamine, but I communicated to the patient and his physician the need of a psychotherapeutic approach once the drug had completed its action, which would be in 3 months.

Sessions 2–6

After patient assessment and reading the diary brought by the patient, a cognitive behavioral strategy is formulated. This may encompass both exposure and cognitive restructuring. Exposure consists of homework exposure only. An exposure strategy is planned with the patient, based on the list of situations outlined in the diary. The therapist writes an assignment per day in the diary, following graded exposure logic [19]. The patient assigns a score from 0 to 100 for each homework assignment. At the following visit, the therapist reassesses the homework done and discusses the next steps, and/or problems in compliance which may have ensued.

Cognitive restructuring follows the format of Beck et al. [20] and is based on the introduction of the concept of automatic thoughts (second session) and of observer interpretation (beginning in the third session), and by the use of macroanalysis (as described in Chapter 4). The latter establishes a relationship among syndromes (the majority of patients with depression do not qualify for one, but for several DSM disorders [7]) and problems on the basis of where treatment should begin in the first place.

The problems which may be objects of cognitive restructuring strictly depend on the material offered by the patient. They may encompass insomnia (sleep hygiene instructions are added), hypersomnia, diminished energy and concentration, residual hopelessness, reentry problems (diminished functioning at work, avoidance, and procrastination), lack of assertiveness and self-care, perfectionism, and unrealistic self-expectations.

What emerges in Mike's case is the fact that his workload exceeds his possibilities, which seems to be unusual in his position as a county clerk in a small town. The city mayor trusts him and relies on him for doing things also in areas that do not pertain to his job description. Additionally, his colleagues frequently ask him for help and he is unable to say no. Mike understands that this is not good for him, but is unable to do otherwise. When through CBT he learns to say 'no' to his colleagues (assertiveness training) and to endorse this attitude consistently, a significant degree of distress ensues, linked to perceived disapproval by others. Cognitive restructuring yields a decrease in distress, but only to a certain degree.

Sessions 7–10

WBT is introduced in the 7th session with the modalities described in Chapter 13. One of the aims of therapy is also that of making the patient aware of allo-

Table 4. Areas that need to be explored for the determination of allostatic overload

Recent life events	Did any of the following happen to you in the past year: death of a family member or close friend, separation, recent change of job, moving, financial difficulties, legal problems, or beginning of a new relationship?
Chronic stress	Do you feel under pressure at work? Do you get along with your colleagues? Do you get along with your spouse/partner or other family members? Do you feel tension at home? Has any close relative been seriously ill in the past year? Were you subjected to mobbing?
Environmental mastery	Do you often feel overwhelmed by the demands of everyday life? Do you often feel you cannot make it?
Sleep	Does it take a long time to fall asleep? Is sleep restless? Do you wake up too early and are not able to go back to sleep?
Somatization	Do you feel tired or a lack of energy? Dizziness? Breathing difficulties? Stomach, bowel pain? Other symptoms?
Psychological distress	Do you feel irritable? Sad or depressed? Tense or 'wound up'?

static loads (i.e., chronic and often subtle life stresses that exert harmful consequences on the individual over a certain amount of time). Examples may be excessive workload, unawareness of the longer time that an increasing age requires for recovering from demanding days, inability to protect oneself from requests which exceed the potential of the individual, and inappropriate sleeping habits [21]. The concept of allostatic overload [21] indicates that external demands exceed the capability of the individual to cope (table 4).

Such awareness (and the resulting lifestyle implementation) are pursued in all phases of psychotherapy, but particularly with WBT. Patients are given instructions in their diaries as to this implementation. WBT allows Mike to realize how his lack of autonomy leads his workmates consistently to take advantage of him, resulting in a workload that, because of its diverse nature, leads to significant stress and increases work hours. The patient accepts the situation by virtue of his low degree of self-acceptance. He claims that this is the way he is, but at the same time he is dissatisfied with himself and chronically irritable. WBT increases his tolerance to disapproval (table 5).

In the last session, Mike is able to make the following remark: 'Now my workmates say that I have changed and that I have become a bastard. In a way I am

Table 5. Mike's well-being diary

Situation	Well-being	Interrupting thoughts and/or behaviors	Observer
George has not finished his work and the mayor asks me to complete it, but I am able to say it is too much for me.	Eventually I can go back home at a decent time and enjoy my family.	The mayor was very disappointed and probably the job was important. I have been selfish.	If George does not do his job, it is not my responsibility. The mayor should make him work and confront him with his responsibilities.

sorry since I have always tried to be helpful and kind to people. But in another way I am happy, because it means that, for the first time in my life, I have been able to protect myself.' Fluvoxamine was tapered and discontinued during psychotherapy. The patient had no further relapse at the 10-year follow-up while being drug-free.

The clinical picture illustrates how an initial feeling of well-being (being helpful to others) identified in the patient's diary was likely to lead to overwhelming distress. Its appraisal and the resulting change in behavior initially led to more distress, but then yielded a lifestyle modification and, hence, a lasting remission [22].

Drug Tapering and Discontinuation

There is a tendency to protract drug treatment for long periods of time, with the assumption that it may be protective against relapse. Evidence from both meta-analyses of randomized controlled trials [23, 24] and naturalistic studies [25, 26] have questioned such views. In these latter investigations, early discontinuers of antidepressant drugs have a better prognosis than those who continue pharmacological treatment. An additional vexing problem is the frequent occurrence of loss of clinical effect in patients who initially responded to the medications [4]. Finally, a negative aspect of long-term antidepressant drug treatments is concerned with the side effects of antidepressant drugs, particularly those that ensue with selective serotonin reuptake inhibitors (SSRI) [27], such as high rates of sexual dysfunction, bleeding (in particular gastrointestinal), weight gain (after initial weight loss), risk of fracture and osteoporosis, and hyponatremia [27]. Sequential treatment provides a unique opportunity for antidepressant drug tapering and discontinuation. In fact, it offers the opportunity to monitor the patient in one of the most delicate aspects of treatment. In the original studies [16, 17], antidepressant drugs were mainly tricyclics and were decreased at the rate of 25 mg of amitriptyline or its equivalents every other week. When SSRI are involved, it is better to have more gradual tapering.

With tricyclic antidepressants, it is important to warn the patient that he or she should not perceive 'steps' (as one patient defined them) in this tapering (i.e., patients should not perceive substantial differences in their sleep, energy, mood, or appetite from 200 mg of amitriptyline per day to 175 mg). If they do, the appropriateness of tapering the antidepressant drug should be questioned. Indeed, in the original studies, drug discontinuation could not take place in a few patients.

'Steps' are very frequent with SSRI, venlafaxine, and duloxetine [4]. They are withdrawal reactions that have been disguised as 'discontinuation syndromes', with the aim to avoid any hint of a potential for dependence from SSRI, venlafaxine, and duloxetine that may affect marketing. These withdrawal syndromes may also occur during tapering and are characterized by a broad range of somatic symptoms (e.g., headache, dizziness, fatigue, diminished appetite, sleep disturbances, and flu-like symptoms) and psychological distress (e.g. agitation, anxiety, dysphoria, and confusion) [28, 29]. These reactions are particularly pronounced with paroxetine and may persist for months or even years after medication discontinuation, leading to what have been defined as 'persistent postwithdrawal disorders' [28, 29].

The benefits of the sequential approach in terms of relapse risk have been maximal when drug discontinuation by slow tapering was achieved [30]. The sequential format offers an ideal opportunity to support the patient psychologically when withdrawal syndromes (despite slow tapering, particularly with SSRI) do occur.

At times, patients are fearful of drug discontinuation. It is then helpful to emphasize that a drug-free status is a step forward in therapy and may be associated with an increased quality of life. It is thus a sign of progress. Antidepressant drugs may be prescribed again if they are needed, when prodromal symptoms of mood deterioration occur, and patients should be reassured about this possibility which is always available.

Table 6. Steps for implementing the sequential approach in depression

1	Careful assessment of the patient 3 months after starting antidepressant drug treatment, with special reference to residual symptoms
2	CBT for residual symptoms, including cognitive restructuring and/or homework exposure
3	Tapering of antidepressant drug treatment at the slowest possible pace
4	Addition of well-being-enhancing therapy and lifestyle modification
5	Discontinuation of antidepressant drugs
6	Careful assessment of the patient 1 month after drug discontinuation

The Efficacy of Sequential Treatment

The sequential approach consists of the application of pharmacotherapy to the acute phase of depression and of psychotherapy in its residual phase. There are two major variants of the sequential model. One consists of continuation of drug treatment during the residual phase. The other involves tapering and discontinuation of antidepressant drugs during psychotherapy. This latter model is the one that is presented here and summarized in table 6. When antidepressant drugs have been discontinued and psychotherapy has been completed, it is important to reassess the patient carefully and to evaluate whether residual symptoms are still present. The Clinical Interview for Depression (CID) [18] is a very useful tool for this purpose.

In this model, psychotherapy addresses only problems and symptoms that were unaffected by drug treatment. Second-line psychotherapy can thus be briefer and more targeted than psychotherapy applied in the initial phase. It requires motivation by the patient and availability of competent therapists. The addition of WBT is supported by research suggesting that impairment of well-being is a strong risk factor for depression in longitudinal studies [31] and is found also in remitted patients with recurrent depression [32].

The sequential model in both variants (drug continuation/discontinuation) was found to yield long-term benefits in terms of enduring remission compared to control conditions, as was substantiated by a meta-analysis on several studies performed by Jenny Guidi, Elena Tomba, and myself [30], including some recent investigations [33–37]. One of these investigations, by Stangier et al. [36], used WBT.

What if the patient has a relapse after antidepressant drug discontinuation, despite doing well in psychotherapy? A lot of care should be exercised in determining whether a true reemergence of the symptoms of a major depressive disorder has occurred or whether the patient is simply going through a difficult life phase. Booster sessions of psychotherapy may be appropriate in this latter case. If a relapse has indeed occurred, new administration of antidepressant drugs is warranted. A general indication is to use the same drug that was found to yield remission in the initial episode [4]. An abridged version of the sequential model can be repeated. I generally tell my patients, 'We should try to see together what went wrong and why. We still have the possibility to learn how we can do better.' There are patients, however, for whom discontinuation of antidepressant drugs is simply not feasible and long-term treatment is indicated [4].

There is also the possibility that an antidepressant drug no longer works although it was successful earlier. We have documented this occurrence in our studies concerned with the sequential model [38, 39]. It was a relatively rare event; however, in trials and naturalistic studies where only drug treatment is administered, it may occur in about one third of the patients [4]. We do not really know what to do in such cases because there is so little research on these topics (a perfect example of the censorship operated by special interest groups in terms of scientific priorities, publishing, and grant access). In these cases, psychiatrists often start to switch drugs, add new compounds, and attempt various combinations. The failure of this strategy was documented, but not emphasized as it should have been [40], in a trial involving thousands of patients, the Sequenced Treatment Alternatives to Relieve Depression (STAR*D) Study [41]. Patients who did not respond to initial treatment with an SSRI were submitted to sequential steps involving switching, augmentation, and combination strategies [41]. The rates of relapse increased after each treatment step and there were refractory states characterized by low remission, high relapse, and high intolerance rates [41]. This trial was concerned with patients who did not respond to initial treatment [42], and while they were not necessarily representative of the patients who had responded, the lessons have far-reaching implications [40].

We reported the case of a depressed patient who had responded well to an antidepressant drug, and the medication was then tapered and discontinued [43]. Three months later depression came back, but this time the same medication that was given the first time did not work. After some pharmacological attempts, the sequential combination of CBT and WBT was performed. She got better and stayed well (I now have a 12-year follow-up with no relapses and psychotropic medications). Interestingly, since the mechanisms of oppositional tolerance with antidepressant drugs may involve the hypothalamic-pituitary-adrenal axis [40], we also measured 24-hour urinary free cortisol, which provides an overall assessment of the production of cortisol. The hypothalamic-pituitary-adrenal axis was normalized by CBT/WBT [43]. Future research may disclose whether WBT has a place in treatment resistance in depression.

Indeed, two other interesting cases were reported in the Netherlands by Peter Meulenbeek, Lieke Christenhusz, and Ernst Bohlmeijer [44]. One involved a patient with depression that was refractory to both pharmacological treatment and CBT, and was successfully treated with WBT. In the other case, WBT was applied to a patient with DSM dysthymia and yielded remission.

Loss of Clinical Effect during Long-Term Treatment with Antidepressant Drugs

As I have discussed before, despite the use of a sequential approach aimed at antidepressant drug discontinuation, there are patients who need to take medications indefinitely. The majority of depressed patients never have a real chance to get appropriate psychotherapy for their mood disturbances. If these patients try to stop their medications, relapse may occur or (if they take SSRI, venlafaxine, and duloxetine which induce dependence [28, 29, 40]) withdrawal symptoms mixed to residual depressive symptomatology may emerge. Therefore, they have to come back to the medication. However, patients may encounter problems even when they never stop antidepressant drugs. Loss of efficacy of antidepressant drugs in long-term treatment of depression is a problem that increases with the duration of treatment (from 23% within 1 year to 34% within 2 years, and to 45% within 3 years) [45].

This problem is generally conceived in pharmacological terms [40]. However, four decades ago, Paykel and Tanner [46] found that relapse in depression was frequently preceded by life events and antidepressant maintenance treatment had little effect on relapse. A number of pharmacological strategies have been suggested for addressing loss of antidepressant efficacy, but with limited success [40]. Ten patients with recurrent depression who relapsed while taking antidepressant drugs were randomly assigned to a dose increase or to a sequential combination of CBT and WBT [47]. Four out of 5 patients responded to a larger dose, but all relapsed again on that dose by the 1-year follow-up. Four out of 5 patients responded to psychotherapy and only one relapsed. The data suggest that application of WBT may counteract loss of clinical effect during long-term antidepressant treatment. It is conceivable that WBT may restore and maintain remission with antidepressant drugs when response fails or is about to fail. This was a small and preliminary study that should be confirmed by large investigations.

A Positive Look at Depression

A rational use of antidepressant drugs that incorporates all potential benefits and harms consists of targeting their application to only the most severe and persistent cases of depression, limiting their use to the shortest possible duration. Unfortunately, when we stretch their original indications (treatment of the acute episode) and we prolong treatment over 6–9 months, we may recruit phenomena such as tolerance, episode acceleration, and paradoxical effects [8]. This may sound depressing, but there is a better message from psychotherapy research and the use of the sequential model. Depression can be defeated and for good.

Often, while experiencing the pain of depression, patients ask me, 'Will I ever be again the person I was before?' My answer is, 'I hope not. You should become much better and learn from the experience.'

References

1 Judd LL: The clinical course of unipolar major depressive disorders. Arch Gen Psychiatry 1997;54:989–991.
2 Fava GA: Subclinical symptoms in mood disorders. Psychol Med 1999;29:47–61.
3 Fournier JC, DeRubeis RJ, Hollon SD, Dimidjian S, Amsterdam JD, Shelton RC, Fawcett J: Antidepressant drug effects and depression severity: a patient-level meta-analysis. JAMA 2010;303:47–53.
4 Fava GA: Rational use of antidepressant drugs. Psychother Psychosom 2014;83:197–204.
5 Paykel ES, Hollyman JA, Freeling P, Sedgwick P: Predictors of therapeutic benefit from amitriptyline in mild depression: a general practice placebo-controlled trial. J Affect Disord 1988;14:83–95.
6 Offidani E, Fava GA, Tomba E, Baldessarini RJ: Excessive mood elevation and behavioral activation with antidepressant treatment of juvenile depressive and anxiety disorders: a systematic review. Psychother Psychosom 2013;82:132–141.
7 Fava GA, Tomba E: New modalities of assessment and treatment planning in depression. CNS Drugs 2010;24:453–465.

8 Fava GA: Long-term treatment with antidepressant drugs: the spectacular achievements of propaganda. Psychother Psychosom 2002; 71:127–132.

9 Diagnostic and Statistical Manual of Mental Disorders, ed 5. Arlington, American Psychiatric Association, 2013.

10 Fava GA, Kellner R: Staging: a neglected dimension in psychiatric classification. Acta Psychiatr Scand 1993;87:225–230.

11 Cosci F, Fava GA: Staging of mental disorders: systematic review. Psychother Psychosom 2013;82:20–34.

12 Tomba E, Fava GA: Treatment selection in depression: the role of clinical judgment. Psychiatr Clin North Am 2012;35:87–98.

13 American Psychiatric Association: Practice Guideline for the Treatment of Patients with Major Depressive Disorder, ed 3. Am J Psychiatry 2010;167(suppl):1–118.

14 Perry PJ: Pharmacotherapy for major depression with melancholic features. J Affect Disord 1996;39:1–6.

15 Tomba E: Nowhere patients. Psychother Psychosom 2012;81:69–72.

16 Fava GA, Rafanelli C, Grandi S, Conti S, Belluardo P: Prevention of recurrent depression with cognitive behavioral therapy: preliminary findings. Arch Gen Psychiatry 1998;55: 816–820.

17 Fava GA, Grandi S, Zielezny M, Canestrari R, Morphy MA: Cognitive behavioral treatment of residual symptoms in primary major depressive disorder. Am J Psychiatry 1994;151: 1295–1299.

18 Guidi J, Fava GA, Bech P, Paykel ES: The Clinical Interview for Depression: a comprehensive review of studies and clinimetric properties. Psychother Psychosom 2011;80: 10–27.

19 Marks IM: Fears, Phobias and Rituals: Panic, Anxiety and Their Disorders. New York, Oxford University Press, 1987.

20 Beck AT, Rush AJ, Shaw BF, Emery G: Cognitive Therapy of Depression. New York, Guilford, 1979.

21 Fava GA, Guidi J, Semprini F, Tomba E, Sonino N: Clinical assessment of allostatic load and clinimetric criteria. Psychother Psychosom 2010;79:280–284.

22 Fava GA, Fabbri S: Drug-resistant and partially remitted depression; in Wishman MA (ed): Adapting Cognitive Therapy for Depression. New York, Guilford Press, 2008, pp 110–131.

23 Kaymaz N, van Os J, Loonen AJ, Nolen WA: Evidence that patients with single versus recurrent depressive episodes are differentially sensitive to treatment discontinuation: a meta-analysis of placebo-controlled randomized trials. J Clin Psychiatry 2008;69:1423–1436.

24 Viguera AC, Baldessarini RJ, Friedberg J: Discontinuing antidepressant treatment in major depression. Harv Rev Psychiatry 1998; 5:293–306.

25 Gardarsdottir H, van Geffen EC, Stolker JJ, Egberts TC, Heerdink ER: Does the length of the first antidepressant treatment episode influence risk and time to a second episode? J Clin Psychopharmacol 2009;29:69–72.

26 Gardarsdottir H, Egberts TC, Stolker JJ, Heerdink ER: Duration of antidepressant drug treatment and its influence on risk of relapse/recurrence: immortal and neglected time bias. Am J Epidemiol 2009;170:280–285.

27 Moret C, Isaac M, Briley M: Problems associated with long-term treatment with selective serotonin reuptake inhibitors. J Psychopharmacol 2009;23:967–974.

28 Belaise C, Gatti A, Chouinard VA, Chouinard G: Persistent postwithdrawal disorders induced by paroxetine, a selective serotonin reuptake inhibitor, and treated with specific cognitive behavioral therapy. Psychother Psychosom 2014;83:247–248.

29 Fava GA, Gatti A, Belaise C, Guidi J, Offidani E: Withdrawal symptoms after selective serotonin reuptake inhibitor discontinuation: a systematic review. Psychother Psychosom 2015;84:72–81.

30 Guidi J, Tomba E, Fava GA: The sequential integration of pharmacotherapy and psychotherapy in the treatment of major depressive disorder: a meta-analysis of the sequential model and a critical review of the literature. Am J Psychiatry 2015, Epub ahead of print.

31 Wood AM, Joseph S: The absence of positive psychological (eudemonic) well-being as a risk factor for depression: a ten year cohort study. J Affect Disord 2010;122:213–217.

32 Risch AK, Taeger S, Brudern J, Stangier U: Psychological well-being in remitted patients with recurrent depression. Psychother Psychosom 2013;82:404–405.

33 Bondolfi G, Jermann F, Van der Linden M, Gex-Fabry M, Bizzini L, Rouget BW, Myers-Arrazola L, Gonzalez C, Segal Z, Aubry JM, Bertschy G: Depression relapse prophylaxis with Mindfulness-Based Cognitive Therapy: replication and extension in the Swiss health care system. J Affect Disord 2010;122:224–231.

34 Godfrin KA, van Heeringen C: The effects of mindfulness-based cognitive therapy on occurrence of depressive episodes, mental health and quality of life: a randomized controlled study. Behav Res Ther 2010;48:738–746.

35 Segal ZV, Bieling P, Young T, MacQueen G, Cooke R, Martin L, Bloch R, Levitan RD: Antidepressant monotherapy vs sequential pharmacotherapy and mindfulness-based cognitive therapy, or placebo, for relapse prophylaxis in recurrent depression. Arch Gen Psychiatry 2010;67:1256–1264.

36 Stangier U, Hilling C, Heidenreich T, Risch AK, Barocka A, Schlösser R, Kronfeld K, Ruckes C, Berger H, Röschke J, Weck F, Volk S, Hambrecht M, Serfling R, Ertkwoh R, Stirn A, Sobanski T, Hautzinger M: Maintenance cognitive-behavioral therapy and manualized psychoeducation in the treatment of recurrent depression: a multicenter prospective randomized controlled trial. Am J Psychiatry 2013;170:624–632.

37 Williams JMG, Crane C, Barnhofer T, Brennan K, Duggan DS, Fennel MJV, Hackmann A, Krusche A, Muse K, Von Rohr IR, Shah D, Crane RS, Eames C, Jones M, Radford S, Silverton S, Sun Y, Wheatherley-Jones E, Whitaker CJ: Mindfulness-based cognitive therapy for preventing relapse in recurrent depression: a randomized dismantling trial. J Consult Clin Psychol 2014;82:275–286.

38 Fava GA, Rafanelli C, Grandi S, Canestrari R, Morphy M: Six-year outcome for cognitive behavioral treatment of residual symptoms in major depression. Am J Psychiatry 1998;155:1443–1445.

39 Fava GA, Ruini C, Rafanelli C, Finos L, Conti S, Grandi S: Six-year outcome of cognitive behavior therapy for prevention of recurrent depression. Am J Psychiatry 2004;161:1872–1876.

40 Fava GA, Offidani E: The mechanisms of tolerance in antidepressant action. Prog Neuropsychopharmacol Biol Psychiatry 2011;35:1593–1602.

41 Rush AJ, Trivedi MH, Wisniewski SR, Nierenberg AA, Stewart JW, Warden D, Niederehe G, Thase ME, Lavori PW, Lebowitz BD, McGrath PJ, Rosenbaum JF, Sackeim HA, Kupfer DJ, Luther J, Fava M: Acute and longer-term outcomes in depressed outpatients requiring one or several treatment steps: a STAR*D report. Am J Psychiatry 2006;163:1905–1917.

42 Carvalho AF, Berks M, Hyphantis TN, McIntyre R: The integrative management of treatment-resistant depression: a comprehensive review and perspectives. Psychother Psychosom 2014;83:70–88.

43 Sonino N, Fava GA: Tolerance to antidepressant treatment may be overcome by ketoconazole. J Psychiatr Res 2003;37:171–173.

44 Meulenbeek P, Christenhusz L, Bohlmeijer E: Well-Being Therapy in the Netherlands. Psychother Psychosom 2015;84:316–317.

45 Williams N, Simpson AN, Simpson K, Nahas Z: Relapse rates with long-term antidepressant drug therapy: a meta-analysis. Hum Psychopharmacol 2009;24:401–408.

46 Paykel ES, Tanner J: Life events, depressive relapse and maintenance treatment. Psychol Med 1976;6:481–485.

47 Fava GA, Ruini C, Rafanelli C, Grandi S: Cognitive behavior approach to loss of clinical effect during long-term antidepressant treatment: a pilot study. Am J Psychiatry 2002;159:2094–2095.

Chapter 15
Mood Swings

Fluctuations of mood appear to be common in the general population [1]. One could view rapid and apparently unjustified changes in mood as subclinical manifestations of one of the most serious and invalidating psychiatric illnesses, bipolar disorder. Originally conceived as the alternation of severe mania and depression ('manic-depressive psychosis'), in recent decades it has broadened its boundaries. There are advantages and disadvantages with this type of approach. The main advantage is to extend the benefits of treatment (mainly pharmacological) to those subjects who would otherwise be neglected. The disadvantage is to conceptualize a wide range of behaviors as pathological and in need of medication [2]. What happened to the misuse of the diagnosis of bipolar disorder in childhood and adolescence leading to largely inappropriate drug use is a sad reminder of a trend that has discredited the image of psychiatry [3].

An alternative approach is to consider that stability of mood is not part of the human existence. If in the morning I listen to the news and hear what the Italian government is planning to do, a bad mood ensues. If I forget about the government later in the morning, my mood improves. The best time for me is when there is no government in Italy and I (as a fool each time) can hope that some decent people will be appointed and something good can be accomplished in this wonderful country. Is my behavior normal? Not really since the majority of Italian people appear to be quite enthusiastic about their prime ministers. It is understandable, however, if you take a historic and economic perspective.

Table 1. CID reactivity to the social environment [6]

This refers to the changes in mood and symptomatology in direction of either improvement or worsening as a result of environmental circumstances. Assess degree: average if this varies. 'Does what is happening around you make a difference to your depression? Or does it not affect it? Do some things bring it on? If you feel bad, are there things which will make you feel a lot better? Does it come on without any reason? Does it change much or stay the same?'	1 = Absent. Changes due to environment absent or very rare. 2 = Very mild or occasional. 3 = Mild. Nonspecific factors, such as having someone to talk to, produce limited improvement. 4 = Moderate. Such factors or certain more specific situations produce greater improvement or worsening. 5 = Marked. Depression varies to a considerable degree according to situational factors. 6 = Severe. Factors frequently completely remove the depression and precipitate it. 7 = Extreme. The source of the depression is entirely dependent on certain specific situations, being regularly precipitated or entirely removed according to them.

In clinical terms, the challenge may be to explore the boundaries between understandable fluctuations of mood and intense fluctuations without any apparent reason. The diagnosis of cyclothymic disorder seems to provide such a threshold [4]. Even though the concept dates back to the nineteenth century, it has largely been ignored since there are no drugs that were patented for the disorder. It is defined as a chronic mood disorder characterized by transient and mild depressive and hypomanic symptoms over at least 2 years. Hypersomnia alternating with decreased need for sleep, shaky self-esteem, periods of apathy alternating with sharpened and creative thinking, uneven productivity, and uninhibited friendliness followed repeatedly by introverted self-absorption characterize cyclothymic disorder [5]. There may be irritable-angry-explosive attacks leading to considerable social embarrassment. It is also associated with substantial comorbidity (including substance and alcohol abuse, as well as anxiety disorders) [4, 5].

In most of our clinical studies, as I mentioned before, we used Paykel's Clinical Interview for Depression (CID) [6], which is probably the most complete and sensitive observer-rated instrument that is available. Jenny Guidi has worked with this instrument, and she alerted my attention to one item of the scale: reactivity to the social environment (table 1).

It is a very important item which you do not find in similar scales. Looking at the effects of Well-Being Therapy (WBT) on individual items of the CID in patients with depressive and anxiety disorders [6], I realized that reactivity to social environment was often improved, as if impairment in well-being could predispose people to intensive reactions during everyday life. I thus designed a controlled study on the use of the sequential combination of cognitive behavior therapy (CBT)/WBT in cyclothymic disorder compared to clinical management, as described in Chapter 3. The treatment protocol that I am going to describe derives from that study [7]. Indeed, the CBT/WBT combination induced improvement in reactivity to the social environment and observer-rated depressive and manic symptoms significantly more as compared to clinical management. At the 2-year follow-up, only a quarter of the patients who were assigned to CBT/WBT still met the diagnostic criteria for cyclothymia compared to 87% of those treated with clinical management [7].

Assessment

First Two Sessions
Cyclothymic features are often in association with other psychiatric disorders that are frequently the primary cause for seeking treatment [8]. Cyclothymia tends to pass unnoticed unless one specifically looks for it. The type of psychiatric illness that is associated with it very much depends on the characteristics of clinical practice. In the setting of our Affective Disorders Program, we find cyclothymic features in many cases of anxiety disorders [8]. The recognition of these symptoms is very important since a physician is likely to prescribe antidepressant drugs in addition to or in substitution of benzodiazepines when anxiety disturbances are accompanied by sadness and demoralization [9]. Antidepressant drugs may stabilize reactivity to the social environment in the short-term, as during a drug trial [6]. However, they may also propel the disturbances to a bipolar course from the very beginning or at some later point in time (the initial effects of a drug may be different from those that ensue with time) [10]. Cyclothymic features may indicate an increased risk of this behavioral activation.

Let us consider the case of Sarah, a young woman in college who presents the biphasic characterization of cyclothymia (hypersomnia/decreased need to sleep, demoralization/overconfidence, uneven productivity) with social phobia, irrita-

Table 2. Monitoring of distress

Situation	Distress (0–100)	Thoughts
I am at home studying, but I cannot get enough concentration.	70	I will never be able to make it. I am a failure.

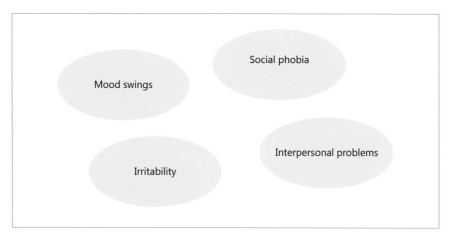

Fig. 1. Macroanalysis of the problems presented by Sarah.

ble-angry-explosive outbursts, and problems with her boyfriend and family. Her primary care physician prescribed antidepressant drugs on two occasions, but she discontinued them since they were making her worse. In a way, I was pleased that she did not take antidepressant drugs since their likelihood to induce hypomania or mania is very high at that age [11]. Sarah's problems are summarized in figure 1 according to macroanalysis.

Upon my request, Sarah started monitoring her episodes of distress (table 2) and developed a hierarchy of phobic situations. When I saw her again 2 weeks later, I decided to tackle the avoidance of social phobia first.

Sessions 3–6
On the basis of macroanalysis of the material that is brought by the patient, in this phase two potential cognitive-behavioral strategies may be used: (1) ex-

Table 3. WBT diary

Situation	Well-being	Interrupting thoughts or behavior	Observer
I was able to study with good profit for 3 hours.	I feel great. I will be able to get rid of this exam quickly.	It will not last. I will screw up everything as I always do.	The time you are studying productively is increasing. There may be loss of concentration, but it is unavoidable.

posure homework for phobic fears (if present), writing each daily assignment in a diary, and (2) introduction of the concept of automatic thoughts and resulting cognitive restructuring. In the case of Sarah I used both strategies, to which she commented: 'I now understand there is a reason for my bad temper.'

Sessions 7–10

In this part the therapist introduces WBT and requires monitoring of well-being instead of distress, with the modalities indicated in the abridged form of WBT (Chapter 13). While doing this, Sarah discovered her low tolerance to well-being (table 3). In particular, she has very little notion of transfer of experiences. Her anxiety performance at university does not change over time.

As Akiskal et al. [5] commented, cyclothymic patients seldom relate their moods to concurrent life situations and, even more, to what they think in those situations. Mood swings, particularly irritable-angry-explosive attacks, put a considerable strain on interpersonal relationships and the patients themselves, who cannot predict, from moment to moment, how they will feel. They avoid anxiety-provoking situations as a source of unpredictable reactivity. This undermines their sense of self and feeds the vicious cycle [5]. The sequential combination of CBT/WBT cognitive restructuring with exposure homework related to social fears allowed Sarah to achieve better control of her mood and to improve her relationships with her boyfriend and family. She said at the end of therapy: 'It is not that I do not have my up and downs, but I know how to react to them, smooth their intensity, and make them last shorter.'

Clinical Implications

Cyclothymia tends to persist over time. In our control group which was assigned to clinical management, the majority of patients still had it 2 years later. However, our findings indicate that it is also a treatable condition. Patients may actually learn to decrease their reactivity to environmental stimuli and to recognize the warnings of mood swings. This may occur, however, only if we are successful in decreasing the anxiety in their lives.

Treatment of anxiety, whenever appropriate, preceded the approach to depressive symptomatology. Behavioral strategies (particularly homework exposure) also preceded cognitive restructuring. The last part of treatment (sessions 7–10) involved monitoring of hypomanic episodes and use of WBT. Colom and Vieta [12] outlined a cognitive model of hypomania characterized by the establishment of positive arbitrary inferences that escape critical appraisal, the selection of thoughts that confirm the most favorable hypothesis, an excessive personalization that can lead to self-referential thought, and a tendency to overinclude stimuli [12]. These cognitions lead to the setting of unrealistic dimensions of psychological well-being, as detailed in Chapters 10–12, which clash with reality.

In cyclothymic disorder, hypomanic thoughts tend to be short lived and have little in common with dimensions of well-being such as environmental mastery, positive relations with others, and self-acceptance. The cognitive restructuring engendered by WBT thus allows the substitution of hypomanic automatic thoughts with sustained feelings of well-being. Even in the manic phases of bipolar disorder, self-esteem has been found to be low [13] and expansiveness and grandiosity may reflect an attempt on the part of the patient to behaviorally offset the covert low levels of well-being [14].

Subclinical fluctuations of mood are the rule in treated bipolar patients and occur in the prodromal phase of illness [15]. It is conceivable, although yet to be tested, that the sequential combination of CBT and WBT that has been used in cyclothymic disorder [7] may yield more enduring effects in terms of relapse rate of remitted bipolar disorder compared to current psychotherapeutic strategies [16]. A pilot investigation on CBT management of residual symptoms in patients with bipolar disorder who relapsed while on lithium prophylaxis [17] was promising in this sense, even though it did not employ WBT.

The goals of the approach we have described are much more ambitious than the customary key themes of the literature on bipolar disorder (psychoeducation, medication adherence, lifestyle regularity, and relapse prevention) that are simply geared to complementing medications. I believe that a positive evaluation of one's self, a sense of continued growth and development, the belief that life is purposeful and meaningful, the possession of quality relations with others, the capacity to manage effectively one's life, and a sense of self-determination, which constitute the bulk of the WBT approach, may also be useful targets for the treatment of bipolar disorder, in addition to mood-stabilizing pharmacological treatment.

References

1 Merikangas KR, Akiskal HS, Angst J, Greenberg PE, Hirschfeld RM, Petukhova M, Kessler RC: Lifetime and 12-month prevalence of bipolar spectrum disorder in the National Comorbidity Survey replication. Arch Gen Psychiatry 2007;64:543–552.

2 Batstra L, Frances A: Holding the line against diagnostic inflation in psychiatry. Psychother Psychosom 2012;81:5–10.

3 Whitaker R: Anatomy of an Epidemic: Magic Bullets, Psychiatric Drugs and the Astonishing Rise of Mental Illness in America. New York, Crown Publishers, 2010.

4 Baldessarini RJ, Vázquez G, Tondo L: Treatment of cyclothymic disorder: commentary. Psychother Psychosom 2011;80:131–135.

5 Akiskal HS, Khan MK, Scott-Strauss A: Cyclothymic temperamental disorders. Psychiatr Clin North Am 1979;2:527–554.

6 Guidi J, Fava GA, Bech P, Paykel ES: The Clinical Interview for Depression: a comprehensive review of studies and clinimetric properties. Psychother Psychosom 2011;80: 10–27.

7 Fava GA, Rafanelli C, Tomba E, Guidi J, Grandi S: The sequential combination of cognitive behavioral treatment and well-being therapy in cyclothymic disorder. Psychother Psychosom 2011;80:136–143.

8 Tomba E, Rafanelli C, Grandi S, Guidi J, Fava GA: Clinical configuration of cyclothymic disturbances. J Affect Disord 2012;139:244–249.

9 Baldwin DS, Allgulander C, Bandelow B, Ferre F, Pallanti S: An international survey of reported prescribing practice in the treatment of patients with generalised anxiety disorder. World J Biol Psychiatry 2012;13:510–516.

10 Fava GA, Offidani E: The mechanisms of tolerance in antidepressant action. Prog Neuropsychopharmacol Biol Psychiatry 2011;35: 1593–1602.

11 Offidani E, Fava GA, Tomba E, Baldessarini RJ: Excessive mood elevation and behavioral activation with antidepressant treatment of juvenile depressive and anxiety disorders: a systematic review. Psychother Psychosom 2013;82:132–141.

12 Colom F, Vieta E: Sudden glory revisited: cognitive contents of hypomania. Psychother Psychosom 2007;76:278–288.

13 Winters KC, Neale JM: Mania and low self-esteem. J Abnorm Psychol 1985;94:282–290.

14 Johnson FN: Different treatment modalities for recurrent bipolar affective disorders. Psychother Psychosom 1986;46:13–22.

15 Fava GA: Subclinical symptoms in mood disorder. Psychol Med 1999;29:47–61.

16 Miklowitz DJ: Adjunctive psychotherapy for bipolar disorder. Am J Psychiatry 2008;165: 1408–1419.

17 Fava GA, Bartolucci G, Rafanelli C, Mangelli L: Cognitive-behavioral management of patients with bipolar disorder who relapsed while on lithium prophylaxis. J Clin Psychiatry 2001;62:556–559.

Chapter 16
Generalized Anxiety Disorder

There are many people who report that they have felt anxious and nervous all their lives. If excessive anxiety and worry exceed a certain clinical threshold, generalized anxiety disorder (GAD) occurs [1]. The disturbance should take place almost every day for at least 6 months, encompassing symptoms such as restlessness, fatigue, difficulty concentrating, irritability, muscle tension, and difficulty falling asleep [1]. Further, the individual finds considerable problems in controlling worries [2]. The diagnostic criteria are based on these symptoms. However, what is probably the most peculiar clinical characteristic (the inability to relax) is not part of the description. These patients never stop worrying. The things that they dread seldom happen. But their life is ruined.

Andy is a college student for whom each exam was a source of terrible anxiety. Anxiety never decreased during his studies (certainly, the concept of transfer of experiences was not familiar to him). It indeed increased before discussion of his Master's thesis. After he successfully passed the final exam, he started worrying about his forthcoming graduation party. He came to me saying: 'I understand that the party is nothing important. But I worry. Does this mean I am condemned to worry and can never have a good moment in my life? Is there something I can do, aside from taking pills?'

In many cases, GAD is associated with other mental disorders (e.g., depression, agoraphobia) and treatment generally follows that of the associated distur-

Table 1. Distress diary

Situation	Distress (0–100)	Thoughts and behaviors

bance [3]. Macroanalysis is a helpful method for establishing treatment priorities in this clinical context. However, in other cases no other associated mental disorder can be found, which was the case for Andy.

Cognitive behavior therapy (CBT) is the treatment of choice for GAD devoid of comorbidities; it is associated with considerable short- and long-term improvements [2]. Drug treatment is also likely to yield relief, but the results are limited to the time of its administration [4]. Contrary to common beliefs among physicians, benzodiazepines are better or as effective as antidepressant drugs, as a member of our research group, Emanuela Offidani, found in a meta-analysis [4–6]. GAD tends to be chronic and unremitting. The goal of treatment should not simply be a decrease of symptoms and worries, but restoration of normal function. For this reason Chiara Rafanelli and I designed a study to compare standard CBT against the sequential combination of CBT and Well-Being Therapy (WBT) [7]. As described in Chapter 3, this latter psychotherapeutic strategy was found to be significantly superior, both after treatment and at follow-up [7]. The following protocol is derived from that controlled study and was improved over the years in clinical practice. It should be implemented only after a careful initial evaluation, as described in Chapter 4. This protocol does not describe the management of concurrent pharmacotherapy since this issue is dealt with in detail in the next chapter.

Session 1

The object of this session is to emphasize the collaborative nature of the therapist/patient relationship and the importance of self-therapy in this context. The self-observation diary is introduced, with a very simple initial task: monitoring the episodes where distress was particularly intense, as suggested in table 1.

Table 2. Goals of session 1

1	Getting a patient's account of how he/she feels, current and past distress, and treatment history
2	Providing information about the structure and modalities of the 8-session course of psychotherapy
3	Establishing a first communication channel and building the basis of a therapeutic alliance
4	Introducing the concept of self-therapy
5	Giving the first homework assignment (diary)

In this phase the therapist refrains from explaining the cognitive model [2] or from making reference to psychological well-being. Elicitation of the patient's understanding of anxiety and its somatic consequences is performed. The first session offers, in fact, the opportunity to learn about the patient's current problems and past treatment history, which may include both pharmacotherapy and psychotherapy. The patient is asked to report in a structured diary the circumstances surrounding the most acute episodes of anxiety, rated on a scale of 0–100, with 0 being absence of anxiety and 100 panic (table 1). The patient is also asked to report thoughts or behaviors that occurred at the time of these anxiety attacks.

The patient is asked to come back in 2 weeks with the diary. The goals of the first session are outlined in table 2.

Session 2

As discussed in Chapter 6, when the patient comes back, a wide range of possibilities occur. If material is presented, no matter how much and in what form, the patient is praised for the collaboration. If no material is brought in, the session is dedicated to exploring the current situation, resistances, difficulties, and misunderstandings; any further development is postponed to the subsequent session. The clinician reviews the diary of the patient. The concept of 'automatic thoughts' is then introduced [2]. The first task is to 'catch' them. After they have been properly identified (and only then), instructions will be given to provide a contrast, slow them down, and reduce the feeling of uncontrollability that accompanies anxiety episodes. Particular attention is paid to the examples that

Table 3. Goals of session 2

1	Checking how the 2 weeks went for the patient in general
2	Review of the diary and the difficulties related to its completion
3	Introducing the concept of automatic thoughts
4	Identifying avoidant behavior
5	Continuing the homework assignments (diary, graded exposure homework if appropriate)

the patient may have provided and to the commonalities between situations in terms of context and types of cognition involved. The patient is encouraged to report automatic thoughts in his/her diary as soon as possible after the anxiety attack. Questions such as 'What was the first thing that went through your mind when you started feeling anxious?' or 'What was your main concern in that situation?' may be helpful. Attention is also dedicated to behaviors that might have occurred during or following episodes of anxiety, with special reference to avoidance patterns [2].

The patient is then asked to continue the diary, with the format outlined in table 1, but with a specific search for automatic thoughts. If avoidance is identified, graded exposure homework is assigned. The patient is asked to come back in 2 weeks.

The goals of the second session are described in table 3.

Session 3

During this session the therapist reviews the homework assignment and praises the patient for recording automatic thoughts and for exposure homework if appropriate. The therapist reviews with the patient the concept of automatic thought and the often associated distorted quality. A column in the diary related to observer's interpretation (what another person would think in the same situation) is introduced (table 4). The therapist starts writing examples of observer's interpretations related to the material presented by the patient.

The patient is thus encouraged to develop alternative perspectives, decatastrophizing fears and gathering evidence [2]. Cognitive errors are identified

Table 4. Distress diary

Situation	Distress (0–100)	Interfering thoughts and/or behaviors	Observer

Table 5. Goals of session 3

1	Checking how the 2 weeks went in general
2	Review of the distress diary, with special reference to identification of automatic thoughts
3	Development of alternative interpretations to automatic thoughts and introduction of the observer's interpretation column
4	Monitoring and enhancing exposure homework as appropriate
5	Continuing with homework assignments (identification of automatic thoughts, column of observer's interpretation, exposure homework)

and modified. The patient is asked to continue the diary and is encouraged to write his/her own observer's interpretations. The patient is asked to come back in 2 weeks. The goals of the third session are outlined in table 5.

Session 4

The clinician praises the patient for the work done and, using a collaborative approach, continues employing techniques in the session to address cognitive errors and undue avoidance. The therapist reviews the diary, with special attention to observer's interpretation, and completes, with the help of the patient, the sections that are missing or deficient. The patient is encouraged to respond immediately to automatic thoughts. Praise is given for efforts that were made by the patient to conduct 'self-therapy'. If it appears that the patient did not go beyond the data collection step, the clinician collaboratively troubleshoots what may have served as obstacles.

In the case of Andy, which was described at the beginning of this chapter, the following aspects of anxious thinking emerged:

Table 6. Goals of session 4

1	Checking how the 2 weeks went in general
2	Review of the distress diary, with special reference to observer's interpretations
3	Encouragement of in vivo interventions of self-therapy, both in terms of contrasting automatic thoughts and avoidance/escape behavior
4	Continuing with homework assignments (identification of automatic thoughts, column of observer's interpretation, exposure homework)

- High threat likelihood (a bad outcome is the most likely possibility, e.g., 'It will certainly go wrong')
- Exaggerated threat severity (anticipating the worst possible outcome) with dichotomic thinking (e.g., 'If I do not make it, I will be fired at once')
- Feelings of inadequacy (e.g., 'I cannot cope with what I am expected to do')

Such aspects were precipitated by the fact that Andy had recently started a postgraduation internship in a firm and was for the first time confronted with the work environment.

The patient is encouraged to continue his/her homework and is told that it is not easy to break well-established habits and ways of thinking. It is possible only with prolonged efforts. The patient is asked to come back in 2 weeks.

The goals of the fourth session are outlined in table 6.

Sessions 5–8

The articulation of the WBT part of the sequential combination that begins with session 5 is the one that is presented in the abridged, post-CBT form of WBT described in Chapter 13. Particular attention, however, is necessary in session 5, which represents the last session of CBT distress-oriented homework and the introduction of the switch to well-being orientation. One general rule to be applied is that the completion of the steps of the approach that is described is far more important than the sequence that is identified by the number of sessions. In other words, it may not be a good practice to move from one step to the other if the patient has not mastered the previous step. For instance, if a patient has trouble identifying automatic thoughts, it is really of no use to introduce the column of observer's interpretation. Similarly, moving to the WBT part requires

Table 7. Andy's well-being diary

Situation	Well-being (0–100)	Interfering thoughts and/or behaviors	Observer
I was able to handle a new situation at work.	It went well (30).	I did it right, but my lack of competence will come out.	I am learning and getting better day after day. I may do something wrong, but I have all opportunities to correct it.

that the patient has made adequate progress in the CBT section. Otherwise it is better to postpone the WBT intervention because, as in the abridged form presented in Chapter 13, it requires identification of automatic thoughts and development of alternative interpretations.

The addition of WBT to the CBT framework in the setting of GAD may lead to a more comprehensive identification of automatic thoughts than that entailed by the customary monitoring of episodes of distress in cognitive therapy [7]. For instance, an improvement in the perceived perception of managing everyday affairs (environmental mastery) may result in a decrease in pessimistic cognitive distortions related to role functioning. Not surprisingly, procedures to increase self-confidence and to reduce demoralization were included in the anxiety management procedures developed for treating GAD [8]. Interpersonal difficulties were reported as a substantial residual problem after CBT [9]. Emphasis on positive relationships with others and self-acceptance in WBT may improve a patient's failure to understand the give and take of human relationships (with ensuing rigidity and unwillingness to make compromises).

Similarly, overcoming the sense of stagnation (personal growth) and providing a sense of direction (purpose in life) may stimulate self-help and exposure [7]. This excerpt from Andy's well-being diary illustrates these mechanisms (table 7). A full case report provides other helpful insights in these processes [10].

An important suggestion on the role of WBT in anxiety came from a member of our research group, Fiammetta Cosci [11], in a case report. She suggested that patients undergoing cognitive therapy who have difficulties in identifying automatic thoughts may find fewer difficulties with WBT because of the change in the type of monitoring (well-being instead of distress).

Clinical Implications of the Well-Being Therapy Approach to Generalized Anxiety Disorder

The results of our randomized controlled trial on the use of WBT in GAD [7] lent support to the sequential administration of treatment components, i.e., cognitive restructuring and exposure in the first phase and WBT at a subsequent stage. Thus, there are similarities between the sequential use of psychotherapeutic strategies in GAD and the sequential use of pharmacotherapy and psychotherapy to improve recovery in mood disorders [12]. The sample that was selected for our randomized controlled trial did not present with psychiatric comorbidity [7]. It is likely, though yet to be tested, that the sequential use of WBT/CBT may have particular applicability when GAD occurs in the setting of other comorbid conditions, such as mood disorders. A very suitable clinical target may be represented by anxious depression (the coexistence of major depressive disorder and GAD), which shows poor response to antidepressant drugs and represents a major challenge for current psychiatric treatment [3].

References

1 Diagnostic and Statistical Manual of Mental Disorders, ed 5. Arlington, American Psychiatric Association, 2013.

2 Clark DA, Beck AT: Cognitive Therapy of Anxiety Disorders. Science and Practice. New York, Guilford Press, 2010.

3 Fava GA, Tomba E: Treatment of comorbid anxiety disorders and depression; in Emmelkamp PMG, Ehring T (eds): The Wiley Handbook of Anxiety Disorders. Chichester, Wiley, 2014, vol 2, pp 1165–1182.

4 Offidani E, Guidi J, Tomba E, Fava GA: Efficacy and tolerability of benzodiazepines versus antidepressants in anxiety disorders: a systematic review and meta-analysis. Psychother Psychosom 2013;82:355–362.

5 Rickels K: Should benzodiazepines be replaced by antidepressants in the treatment of anxiety disorders? Fact or fiction? Psychother Psychosom 2013;82:351–352.

6 Balon R: Benzodiazepines revisited. Psychother Psychosom 2013;82:353–354.

7 Fava GA, Ruini C, Rafanelli C, Finos L, Salmaso L, Mangelli L, Sirigatti S: Well-Being Therapy of generalized anxiety disorder. Psychother Psychosom 2005;74:26–30.

8 Butler G, Cullington A, Hibbert G, Klines I, Gelder M: Anxiety management for persistent generalised anxiety. Br J Psychiatry 1987; 15:535–542.

9 Borkovec TP, Newman MG, Pincus AG, Lytle R: A component analysis of cognitive behavioral therapy for generalized anxiety disorder and the role of interpersonal problems. J Consult Clin Psychol 2002;70:288–298.

10 Ruini C, Fava GA: Well-being therapy for generalized anxiety disorder. J Clin Psychol 2009;65:510–519.

11 Cosci F: Well-being therapy in a patient with panic disorder who failed to respond to paroxetine and cognitive behavior therapy. Psychother Psychosom 2015;84:318–319.

12 Fava GA, Tomba E: New modalities of assessment and treatment planning in depression. CNS Drugs 2010;24:453–465.

Chapter 17
Panic and Agoraphobia

Agoraphobia is the most common and distressing phobic disorder. Since West-phal's description in 1871, it has been consistently reported in the literature [1].

> The anxiety is at its most intense in enclosed spaces such as shops, vehicles, cinemas, theatres or churches, particularly when the patient finds himself surrounded by a crowd of people. He then begins to feel hot, flustered, tremulous, foolish and panic stricken. Waiting in such crowd or a tube tends to cause mounting anxiety which leads the patient to take flight in fear and embarrassment. When questioned about these experiences some patients describe fear of developing a panic attack or exhibiting anxiety in the presence of others, of fainting or being seen in a helpless or uncontrolled state which they regard as humiliating and embarrassing in the extreme. Once a syncopal attack has occurred the phobias are almost invariably intensified and some patients are wholly incapacitated from shopping or even walking alone in the streets thereafter... Although anxiety is at its most intense if the patient is in a crowded enclosed space, some degree of tension persists during the whole of the time... [2, p 93].

This is the description of agoraphobia in what remains the unsurpassed textbook of psychiatry, the one which was the result of the extraordinary encounter, friendship, and scientific collaboration of William Mayer-Gross, Eliot Slater, and Martin Roth [2].

The phenomenological development of agoraphobia may be categorized according to stages [1, 3, 4]. Table 1 describes such development. The first stage of development involves the presence of predisposing factors, such as genetic vulnerabilities, premorbid personality (in particular dependence and harm avoidance), anxiety sensitivity, and hypochondriacal fears and beliefs [1]. The relative

Table 1. Staging of agoraphobia (modified from Fava et al. [1])

Stage 1	Pre-agoraphobia: presence of anxiety (including health anxiety and anxiety sensitivity) and/or isolated fears and/or personality factors such as dependence and harm avoidance and/or impaired psychological well-being
Stage 2	Agoraphobia: fear of being in places or situations from which escape might be difficult of mild (some avoidance or endurance with distress, but relatively normal lifestyle) or moderate (constricted lifestyle) severity according to DSM-5 criteria
Stage 3	Panic disorder (acute phase): appearance of panic attacks and development of panic disorder (DSM-5); worsening of agoraphobia and anxiety; health anxiety may turn in hypochondriasis and/or disease phobia and/or fear of dying; demoralization and/or major depression may occur
Stage 4	Panic disorder (chronic phase): agoraphobia may become severe (avoidance results in being nearly or completely housebound) according to DSM-5 and hypochondriacal fears and beliefs may accentuate when panic disorder exceeds 6 months; increased liability to major depression

weight of these factors may vary from patient to patient and lead to subtle avoidance patterns and ultimately to agoraphobia (stage 2).

In some patients, agoraphobia may be confined to mild or moderate severity (table 1), whereas in other patients these avoidances paint 'the individual into a corner when further avoidances are no longer tenable or the life situation no longer allows them, and panic ensues' [5].

Two independent studies [6, 7] found that the majority of 40 patients with panic disorder with agoraphobia experienced prodromal symptoms (agoraphobia, hypochondriasis, generalized anxiety) before the first panic attack. The findings were obtained with considerable methodological precautions: careful dating of symptom onset, rigorous symptom definition by a reliable and validated probe suitable for prodromal and subclinical symptoms, and delay of the interview until the acute disturbance has passed (to minimize distortions of recall). Not surprisingly, the findings were confirmed by subsequent studies, reviewed in detail elsewhere [1].

Prodromal avoidance may thus kindle central noradrenergic neurons in the locus coeruleus, also in conjunction with stressful life events. Panic attacks are likely to induce a considerable worsening of prodromal symptomatology: generalized anxiety may acquire a strong anticipatory connotation, agoraphobia may worsen considerably, and nonspecific health anxiety may turn into severe hypochondriasis and thanatophobia (fear of dying; stage 3).

The duration of panic disorder with agoraphobia may be a predisposing factor for the development of other psychiatric complications, notably depression (stage 4). Stressful life events – together with other factors – may play a role in the development of panic or secondary depression.

This four-stage model has many limitations. It may not apply to all patients with agoraphobia (e.g., patients may develop depression before or at the same time of panic disorder). However, it has heuristic value. It may account for agoraphobia without panic attacks being more frequent than panic disorder with agoraphobia [1]. It may explain why hypochondriacal fears and beliefs as well as anxiety sensitivity were found to improve upon behavioral or drug treatment of agoraphobia with panic attacks, and yet were reported as prodromal symptoms or residual/premorbid traits in recovered patients [1]. Most of all, it may be of value in assessing and understanding the changes induced by psychiatric treatment of panic disorder with agoraphobia.

Exposure in vivo by homework exercises is the treatment of choice of agoraphobia associated with panic disorder [8]. Exposure-based interventions are often associated with other cognitive strategies, even though there is no evidence that additional components (e.g., cognitive restructuring, breathing retraining) improve outcomes compared to exposure alone [8]. Antidepressants and benzodiazepines have also been found to be effective in agoraphobia and panic attacks. The main difference is the duration of clinical effects: homework exposure produces lasting improvements [9], whereas the effects of psychotropic drugs wane after their discontinuation [10]. As I mentioned in the previous chapter, benzodiazepines are significantly more effective compared to antidepressant drugs [10–12], in contrast to what most of the psychiatrists tend to believe. The combination of drugs and psychotherapy was not found to yield additional benefits. Indeed, in two major trials it was found to be detrimental [13, 14].

A major problem in treating agoraphobia which has reached the level of panic is that there is a substantial proportion of patients (at least one third) that does not respond or drops out of treatment [9]. In a controlled trial, with a crossover design, three treatment modalities, namely exposure alone, exposure associated with imipramine, and cognitive therapy supplementing exposure, were compared in a sample of 21 patients with DSM-IV panic disorder and agoraphobia who did not respond to exposure [15]. Twelve of the 21 patients achieved remission (panic-free status) during the trial. This occurred after exposure alone in 8 cases, and the other two modalities had 2 cases each. Three patients dropped out of treatment. Resistance to exposure in panic disorder was found to be associated with lower compliance with regard to exposure homework [15]. Compliance, particularly in behavioral settings, requires endurance and motivation. It was thus conceivable that Well-Being Therapy (WBT) might either complete the degree of improvement afforded by symptom-oriented treatments or increase compliance, or both.

The 6 patients who completed treatment but still suffered from panic attacks were offered a course of WBT, and 3 patients accepted. WBT was associated with the prolongation of exposure in vivo homework [16]. Two of the 3 patients achieved panic-free status. It is obviously very difficult to draw conclusions from this very small trial, which involved only half of the patients who still suffered from panic disorder. A placebo (nonspecific) effect is possible, even though unlikely in patients who had unsuccessfully undergone three consecutive trials. Since the controlled trial had disclosed a significant effect of the time factor [15], the results might have been simply due to prolongation of exposure. However, it is also possible that WBT helped the 2 patients undergoing exposure and increased their compliance as to exposure homework. Indeed, this appeared to have been improved according to the therapist's ratings [16]. Fiammetta Cosci [17] described a case of patient with panic disorder, agoraphobia, and a major depressive episode who failed to respond to paroxetine and cognitive behavior therapy (CBT), but successfully responded to WBT. This patient was unable to identify automatic thoughts by monitoring distress as in cognitive therapy, but was able to do it while monitoring well-being with WBT. Interestingly, after WBT she was able to complete cognitive therapy [17].

These results would not, of course, justify the use of WBT. However, it may be interesting to outline in this chapter a treatment protocol based on the combination of exposure treatment and WBT, which is different from the type of combination I have described in depression, cyclothymia, and generalized anxiety disorder (GAD). As a clinical justification, the use of WBT may be based on the significantly lower levels of psychological well-being that were found in remitted patients with panic disorder and agoraphobia compared to healthy controls matched for sociodemographic variables [18]. Further, there are some suggestions that WBT may also play a role in drug treatment discontinuation in anxiety disturbances such as panic [19], as detailed later in this chapter.

Table 2. Goals of session 1

1	Getting a patient's account of how he/she feels, current and past distress, and treatment history
2	Providing information about the structure and modalities of the 12-session course of psychotherapy
3	Establishing a first communication channel and building the basis of a therapeutic alliance
4	Introducing the concept of self-therapy
5	Giving a first homework assignment

Treatment of Panic Disorder and Agoraphobia

The protocol includes 12 sessions lasting 45 min, once every other week. They are based on behavioral exposure homework, but the last 4 sessions encompass a combination of WBT with exposure. Therapy is based on exposure homework only and feedback from the therapist without therapist-aided exposure. We owe this protocol to the outstanding work of Professor Isaac Marks in London [20]. This protocol has been used by our group in one randomized controlled trial [15] and in two open longitudinal investigations [9, 21].

Session 1

The object of this session is to emphasize the collaborative nature of the therapist/patient relationship and the importance of self-therapy in this context. After getting an account of how the patient feels and treatment history, the therapist asks the patient to report in a diary the situations he/she may fear or feel uncomfortable with and that are avoided or faced with distress. In this phase I refrain from suggesting behavioral tasks or from making reference to the cognitive model (this protocol does not include cognitive restructuring or other related techniques) or to psychological well-being. Elicitation of the patient's understanding of anxiety and its somatic consequences is performed.

Most of the patients take psychotropic drugs at the time of intake. The patients are advised to continue to do so until the time is ripe to get rid of them, which is when a certain degree of remission occurs. The clinician and the patient will decide, in a shared decision, exactly when. The patient is asked to come back in 2 weeks with the diary. Table 2 outlines the goals of the first session.

Table 3. List of situations that are avoided or endured with distress (0–100)

- Going to a mall: 80
- Being downtown: 80
- Crowded environments: 80
- Having a meal outside: 70
- Meeting new people: 80
- Being alone at home: 40

Session 2

As discussed in the previous chapter and in Chapter 6, a wide range of possibilities occur when the patient comes back. If material is presented, the patient is praised for the collaboration. If no material is brought, the session is dedicated to exploring current situations, resistances, difficulties, and misunderstandings, and any further development is postponed to the subsequent session. It is explained to the patient: 'We cannot start working unless you bring the diary.' A patient I had referred for behavioral exposure to a clinical psychologist came back to me after a year and complained, 'You told me it was going to be a brief therapy, but it was not so. We had more than 20 sessions and I am still at the point where I started.' Too bad that it took 18 sessions to convince her to bring the diary.

The clinician reviews the diary of the patient. Let us consider the case of Jill. Jill is a 32-year-old physician who works as a cardiologist in a general hospital. She suffers from panic attacks that occur with a frequency of a couple per month despite the use of self-prescribed sertraline (currently 50 mg/day; previously up to 100 mg/day). Self-prescription of psychotropic drugs is a bad habit physicians have. She has been taking sertraline for 2 years since in cardiology she was taught to prescribe it to any patient who appears to be down after a myocardial infarction, an unsubstantiated practice that is another example of the spectacular achievements of propaganda [22]. Her agoraphobia is subtle, as it often is [1]. She can go to work (a 20-km ride by car each way) every day, but refrains from doing anything different. Her list of situations that are avoided or endured with distress is displayed in table 3. She is single and living alone, something she dislikes but has learned to live with. Her list, as it generally happens, is very partial. I suspect that many more situations are part of the clinical picture and will emerge in due course.

After a first assessment of the diary, I generally use the following story that concerned a patient I had at the beginning of my career.

An adolescent boy had recurrent panic attacks, particularly when he was in his high school. Each time he called parents to bring him back home. The first time I saw him I simply told him that he could not give up so easily (he missed so many days that his continuation of high school was in jeopardy): 'You must try to resist; next time we see each other I will explain you how.' When he came back after 2 weeks he shared the following story. 'I had to go to a department store because I needed to make some purchases. As I got in, the 'concert' started. First with some instruments (palpitations, tremors, muscle tension) I could handle. But when I start feeling unsteady and dizzy, I cannot make it and I have to leave the place.' This is what happened to him in the department store, but he remembered my words ('do not give up at the first symptoms') and stayed. Within a minute the 'concert' had stopped. He was pleased with his accomplishment ('it is easier than I thought'). The day after he was riding his bike to a friend's place, something he was used to doing, when he was suddenly struck by another panic attack. While the visit to the department store was predicted to arouse anxiety, this panic attack was quite unexpected, as it took place in a familiar setting. He was not able to go on and went back home. The distress lasted for hours. He then told me he had understood what his illness was about. 'It is like a dog; if you do not show any fear (even if you are actually frightened) the dog will leave you alone and will not attack you. But, if the dog realizes that you are frightened and that you are planning to escape, the dog will chase you and attack you.

I then explain to the patient that he/she will have to confront the dog and learn to show no fear, no matter how much turmoil is inside. The only help the therapist may give, by knowing 'all the dog's dirty tricks', is to explain the best strategies of exposure. An exposure strategy is indeed planned with the patient. It emphasizes the importance of regular, prolonged exposure to phobic situations and recording this in the diary. The central principle of this treatment is to persuade the patient to reenter the phobic situation and to remain there despite the ensuing anxiety [20]. The harmful consequences of avoidant behavior are emphasized.

The clinician writes the assignment in the diary; these tasks constitute the minimal amount of work. The patient is encouraged to do more. Jill's assignments are reported in table 4. They start from the day of the appointment. These assignments take into consideration the fact that Jill's working day is very long and there seems to be little time for doing something else. Jill is asked to give a 0–100 rating as to the difficulty of each exercise, after completing it.

The goals of session 2 are detailed in table 5.

Sessions 3–7
During these sessions the clinician checks how the time period between sessions went and reviews the homework assigned, including the ratings of the patient. Each assignment is briefly discussed, particularly if there were problems or when the patient did not complete it. Patients are advised of the harmless nature and

Table 4. Jill's homework assignments

Wednesday	Stop in a supermarket on the way home
Thursday	Stop in a department store on the way home
Friday	Take a 10-min walk after dinner
Saturday	Go to the supermarket
Sunday	Take a 20-min walk in the morning
Monday	Stop in a department store on the way home
Tuesday	Stop in a supermarket on the way home
Wednesday	Stop in a bookstore on the way home
Thursday	Take a 20-min walk after dinner
Friday	Stop in a department store on the way home
Saturday	Go shopping downtown
Sunday	Take a 30-min walk
Monday	Stop in a supermarket on the way home
Tuesday	Stop in a bookstore on the way home
Wednesday	Next appointment

Table 5. Goals of session 2

1	Checking how the 2 weeks went for the patient in general
2	Review of the diary and the difficulties related to its completion
3	Homework assignments for the following 2 weeks
4	Explanation of the assignments and encouragement

short-lived features of panic attacks and that panic can only subside after adequate work-up.

Detre and Jarecki [23] described the 'rollback phenomenon' in psychopathology: as the illness remits, it progressively recapitulates, even though in a reverse order, many of the stages and symptoms that were seen during the time it developed. Rifkin et al. [24] found that spontaneous and situational panic attacks remit before agoraphobia both in patients treated with alprazolam and placebo. In one of our studies [21], we reported that after six sessions of behavioral treatment solely directed to agoraphobia, all patients still reported panic attacks against a background of significantly improved agoraphobia. Exposure, however, modified the frequency, duration, and quality of panic attacks. Six further sessions of behavioral treatment induced more improvement of agoraphobia and resulted in abatement of panic attacks in the majority of patients. The phe-

Table 6. Goals of sessions 3–7

1	Checking how the time period between the sessions went
2	Review of the diary and of the difficulties encountered by the patient; praise for homework
3	Homework assignments (exposure to increasingly difficult situations)
4	Explanation of the assignments and encouragement

nomenological sequence that was observed retrospectively for the prodromal symptoms of panic disorder (stages 2–3) was thus confirmed by a prospective observation: a decrease in avoidance by exposure resulted in improvement in agoraphobia and panic, with eventual disappearance of panic, whereas agoraphobia persisted, though to a much lesser degree. The rollback phenomenon is also supported by the fact that in the year before relapse of panic, an increase in agoraphobic avoidance was observed, even though a further increase was found after the relapse of panic [25]. Prodromal symptoms of panic disorder thus tend to transform into residual symptomatology, which in turn may progress to become prodromal symptoms of relapse [26].

The exposure homework that takes place in these early sessions is generally unable to result in disappearance of panic [21]. However, panic attacks become milder, with fewer symptoms, and with a marked reduction in the attempt to escape (the 'dog', the behavioral counterpart of panic attacks that has not received adequate attention [21]). Once the prodromes of panic occur, patients appear to react in a way (fight reaction) different from the one prior to therapy (flight reaction) [21]. Jill reacts with initial denial of her difficulties, but then gets into the struggle and, with ups and downs (I always tell the story of my cast, see Chapter 2), extends her mobility.

Sessions take place every other week. The clinician reviews the material and adds new progressive assignments each time. The technical difficulty is the ability to find intermediate steps among assignments and to identify the subtle hierarchy of fears that each individual patient has.

The goals of sessions 3–7 are outlined in table 6.

Session 8

This is the session when WBT is added to the exposure homework. It differs from previous additions since it does not result in replacement of the first-line ap-

Table 7. Goals of session 8

1	Checking how the time period between the sessions went
2	Review of the exposure diary and of the difficulties encountered by the patient
3	Homework assignments (exposure to increasingly difficult situations)
4	Well-being diary

proach (CBT), but in its augmentation. Unlike what has been suggested in GAD (Chapter 16), such an augmenting approach does not require that the patient has successfully completed the previous steps since WBT may actually act as a motivation to exposure, as was found to apply to treatment-resistant cases [16].

The first part of the session follows the format of the previous ones (sessions 2–7), but the patient is asked to look for new tasks. The patient is thus encouraged to monitor the instances of well-being, as detailed in Chapter 6, in a separate diary and to come back in 2 weeks.

The goals of session 8 are detailed in table 7.

Session 9

As happened to many patients, Jill also reacted to the invitation to monitor well-being as an impossible task ('I never feel well'). Nonetheless, she was able to bring a few instances, particularly when things went smoothly as to her homework. In the meantime, her mobility greatly increased: she took a plane again (after years) and sometimes went away from her hometown on weekends. While the first half of the session is still based on review of behavioral exposure (as in the previous sessions), the second considers the well-being diary. The patient is asked to report thoughts or behaviors that lead to premature termination of well-being, as detailed in Chapter 6. The goals of session 9 are outlined in table 8.

Session 10

Exposure homework leads to the disappearance of panic attacks in the majority of patients [21]. This is indeed what happens in Jill's second half of exposure therapy (sessions 7–12).

Yet, disappointing instances when 'the dog barks again' still take place. Jill was aware that she is still taking sertraline and wondered what would happen without it. I replied that she was taking sertraline also when she had panic attacks, and

Table 8. Goals of session 9

1	Checking how the period between the sessions went
2	Review of exposure diary, with problems and achievements; praise and encouragement
3	Review of the well-being diary; introducing the monitoring of thoughts or behaviors that interrupt well-being
4	Beginning to understand which feelings and experiences make the patient feel better, including optimal experiences
5	Continuing with homework assignments (exposure and well-being diary)

Table 9. Well-being diary

Situation	Well-being (0–100)	Interfering thoughts and/or behaviors
My weekend in Rome really went well and I enjoyed the city.	I start living again; I have made a lot of progress from the beginning (60).	This is not going to last. In a short time I will be back in pain again.

that the drug was certainly not helping her with panic. She then voiced an important worry: 'What you say is possible, but without sertraline I would be depressed and hopeless. I believe I am a weak person who cannot make it without antidepressant drugs.' I told her (let's not forget she is a physician) that antidepressant drugs are unlikely to be more effective than placebo after 2 years [27], and that I would give her a demonstration of my thesis in a short while. In reviewing the well-being diary, instances such as the one depicted in table 9 emerged.

Jill was then introduced to the concept of 'automatic thoughts' and asked to look for them, as explained in Chapter 7. She was also asked to reduce her sertraline from 50 to 25 mg per day. I hoped we would have some luck and that the reduction would not give her trouble with withdrawal symptoms.

The goals of session 10 are detailed in table 10. The review of the exposure part should take no longer than one third of the time. The patient is asked to come back in 2 weeks.

Session 11
Jill is able to work effectively with her well-being diary, to catch automatic thoughts, and to introduce observer's interpretations. The decrease in the dos-

Table 10. Goals of session 10

1	Checking how the period between the sessions went
2	Review of exposure diary, with problems and achievements; praise and encouragement
3	Review of the well-being diary as to automatic thought identification
4	Introduction of the observer's column
5	Continuing with homework assignments (exposure and well-being diary)

Table 11. Jill's well-being diary

Situation	Well-being (0–100)	Interfering thoughts and/or behaviors	Observer
At work I was able to speak for my rights.	It is the first time I am able. I am getting good (80).	It is just a little episode. Your colleagues will take advantage of you as they always do.	It is not an isolated episode. I am growing in all the areas of my life.

age of sertraline did not yield any changes in anxiety or mood. I thought I had some luck and thus decided to discontinue sertraline with the option of prescribing bromazepam, which she had taken in the past when needed. Discussion of automatic thoughts revealed impairments in the dimensions of environmental mastery and interpersonal relationships the patient became aware of. At the same time, she realized her major advances in personal growth, as the example portrayed in table 11 indicates.

Session 11 is divided into an exposure part and a well-being part, as in the previous one. Table 12 summarizes its main goals. Termination of therapy is discussed with opportunities to voice fears and feelings. The patient is asked to come back in 2 weeks.

Session 12
In the last session, the issues related to therapy termination are further explored. Both the exposure and well-being diaries are reviewed. The concept of self-therapy is further reinforced: the patient is expected to work on his or her own. The clinician is always available, by telephone or by appointment, when needed. In any case, he/she would like to see the patient again in a year or so. The goals of

Table 12. Goals of session 11

1	Checking how the period between the sessions went and the feelings of the patient as to the impending therapy termination
2	Review of exposure diary
3	Review of the well-being diary; cognitive restructuring according to the dimensions of psychological well-being
4	Continuing with homework assignments (exposure and well-being diary)

Table 13. Goals of session 12

1	Checking the patient's feeling about ending therapy
2	Review of the well-being diary, underscoring improvements that have occurred in the various areas of well-being and in the amount of distress
3	Discussing difficulties that limited self-therapy with WBT
4	Modulating psychological dimensions of well-being by cognitive restructuring
5	Confirming availability for future "booster" sessions; arranging for follow-up

session 12 are described in table 13. It is emphasized that self-therapy never stops and is a never-ending process of personal growth.

Jill did not have problems with sertraline discontinuation and this reinforced the idea that she could survive without it (a little bit of luck is often the blessing of psychotherapy). She communicated that she wanted to get rid of the 'dog' for good (she felt it was still there) and had decided to go abroad for 6 months: 'I need some change in all areas of my life.' She picked an underdeveloped country and was aware of the challenges she was facing. I met her again after that period (prolonged to 9 months). She was much better than before leaving. She was also planning to change her current job in Italy. 'I am growing', she said smiling.

Psychotropic Drug Discontinuation

In recent years a progressive change in the pharmacotherapy of anxiety disorders has occurred: benzodiazepines have been progressively replaced by antidepressant drugs [in particular selective serotonin reuptake inhibitors (SSRI), venlafaxine, and duloxetine] [10–12]. Such a shift can be considered the most spectacular achievement of propaganda in psychiatry since the evidence indicates that benzodiazepines are more or as effective and have minimal side effects compared to antidepressants [10]. A major drive in the shift was the risk of dependence with benzodiazepines. However, in due course after their introduction, similar and more pronounced problems occurred with most of the newer antidepressants. With Chiara Rafanelli and Elena Tomba, we explored the prevalence of withdrawal symptoms ensuing with gradual tapering of SSRI in patients with panic disorder and agoraphobia [28]. The conditions could be judged to be optimal: all patients had fully remitted upon behavioral treatment and were psychologically prepared for tapering and discontinuation. Much to our surprise, 9 of the 20 patients (45%) experienced a withdrawal syndrome, which subsided within a month in all but 3 patients. These 3 patients all received paroxetine and displayed alternations of worsened mood, fatigue, and emotional instability with trouble sleeping, irritability, and hyperactivity [28].

After the publication of our findings, I received many e-mails from patients who made me aware that these persistent postwithdrawal disorders were much more common than I had thought and alerted me to websites describing them. I decided to ask a friend for help: Professor Guy Chouinard, one of the most important psychopharmacologists who had introduced many drugs into practice. He had reported the phenomenon of persistent postwithdrawal disorder earlier than we did [29]. With the help of other researchers from our group, Carlotta Belaise and Alessia Gatti, and Chouinard's own daughter, Virginie-Ann, websites were critically examined and our clinical material was interpreted [30]. A systematic review of the literature indicates that the term 'discontinuation syndrome' that the pharmaceutical industry had coined for SSRI and serotonin-norepinephrine reuptake inhibitor withdrawal reactions was indeed misleading [31, 32]. How can we help patients overcome these persistent postwithdrawal disorders? With Carlotta Belaise we devised a sequential combination of CBT/WBT that consists of 6–16 weekly sessions and which has been detailed elsewhere [19]. As in the case of Jill, it is important to convey the message that 'there is life after antidepressant drugs' and WBT may be a helpful tool in this freedom path.

References

1 Fava GA, Rafanelli C, Tossani E, Grandi S: Agoraphobia is a disease. Psychother Psychosom 2008;77:133–138.

2 Mayer-Gross W, Slater E, Roth M: Clinical Psychiatry. London, Bailliere Tindall, 1977.

3 Cosci F, Fava GA: Staging of mental disorders. Psychother Psychosom 2013;82:20–34.

4 Fava GA, Mangelli L: Subclinical symptoms of panic disorder: new insights into pathophysiology and treatment. Psychother Psychosom 1999;68:281–289.

5 Furlong FW: Antecedents of 'spontaneous' panic attacks. Am J Psychiatry 1989;146:560.

6 Fava GA, Grandi S, Canestrari R: Prodromal symptoms in panic disorder with agoraphobia. Am J Psychiatry 1988;145:1564–1567.

7 Fava GA, Grandi S, Rafanelli C, Canestrari R: Prodromal symptoms in panic disorder with agoraphobia: a replication study. J Affect Disord 1992;26:85–88.

8 Emmelkamp PMG: Behavior therapy with adults; in Lambert MJ (ed): Bergin and Garfield's Handbook of Psychotherapy and Behavior Change, ed 6. New York, Wiley, 2013, pp 343–392.

9 Fava GA, Rafanelli C, Grandi S, Conti S, Ruini C, Mangelli L, Belluardo P: Long-term outcome of panic disorder with agoraphobia treated by exposure. Psychol Med 2001;31: 891–898.

10 Offidani E, Guidi J, Tomba E, Fava GA: Efficacy and tolerability of benzodiazepines versus antidepressants in anxiety disorders: a systematic review and meta-analysis. Psychother Psychosom 2013;82:355–362.

11 Rickels K: Should benzodiazepines be replaced by antidepressants in the treatment of anxiety disorders? Fact or fiction? Psychother Psychosom 2013;82:351–352.

12 Balon R: Benzodiazepines revisited. Psychother Psychosom 2013;82:353–354.

13 Marks IM, Swinson RP, Başoğlu M, Kuch K, Noshirvani H, O'Sullivan G, Lelliott PT, Kirby M, McNamee G, Sengun S, Wickwire K: Alprazolam and exposure alone and combined in panic disorder with agoraphobia. A controlled study in London and Toronto. Br J Psychiatry 1993;162:776–787.

14 Barlow DH, Gorman JM, Shear MK, Woods SW: Cognitive-behavioral therapy, imipramine, or their combination for panic disorder: a randomized controlled trial. JAMA 2000;283:2529–2536.

15 Fava GA, Savron G, Zielezny M, Grandi S, Rafanelli C, Conti S: Overcoming resistance to exposure in panic disorder with agoraphobia. Acta Psychiatr Scand 1997;95:306–312.

16 Fava GA: Well-being therapy: conceptual and technical issues. Psychother Psychosom 1999; 68:171–179.

17 Cosci F: Well-being therapy in a patient with panic disorder who failed to respond to paroxetine and cognitive behavior therapy. Psychother Psychosom 2015;84:318–319.

18 Fava GA, Rafanelli C, Ottolini F, Ruini C, Cazzaro M, Grandi S: Psychological well-being and residual symptoms in remitted patients with panic disorder and agoraphobia. J Affect Disord 2001;65:185–190.

19 Belaise C, Gatti A, Chouinard V-A, Chouinard G: Persistent postwithdrawal disorders induced by paroxetine, a selective serotonin reuptake inhibitor, and treated with specific cognitive behavioral therapy. Psychother Psychosom 2014;83:247–248.

20 Marks IM: Fears, Phobias and Rituals. New York, Oxford University Press, 1987.

21 Fava GA, Grandi S, Canestrari R, Grasso L, Pesarin F: Mechanisms of change of panic attacks with exposure treatment of agoraphobia. J Affect Disord 1991;22:65–71.

22 Rafanelli C, Sirri L, Grandi S, Fava GA: Is depression the wrong treatment target for improving outcome in coronary artery disease? Psychother Psychosom 2013;82:285–291.

23 Detre TP, Jarecki HG: Modern Psychiatric Treatment. Philadelphia, Lippincott, 1971.

24 Rifkin A, Pecknold JC, Swinson RP, Ballenger JC, Burrows GD, Noyes R, Dupont RL, Lesser I: Sequence of improvement in agoraphobia with panic attacks. J Psychiatr Res 1990;24: 1–8.

25 Fava GA, Zielezny M, Savron G, Grandi S: Long-term effects of behavioural treatment for panic disorder with agoraphobia. Br J Psychiatry 1995;166:87–92.

26 Fava GA, Kellner R: Prodromal symptoms in affective disorders. Am J Psychiatry 1991;148: 823–830.

27 Fava GA: Rational use of antidepressant drugs. Psychother Psychosom 2014;83:197–204.

28 Fava GA, Bernardi M, Tomba E, Rafanelli C: Effects of gradual discontinuation of selective serotonin reuptake inhibitors in panic disorder with agoraphobia. Int J Neuropsychopharmacol 2007;10:835–838.

29 Bhanji NH, Chouinard G, Kolivakis T, Margolese HC: Persistent tardive rebound panic disorder, rebound anxiety and insomnia following paroxetine withdrawal. Can J Clin Pharmacol 2006;13:69–74.

30 Belaise C, Gatti A, Chouinard VA, Chouinard G: Patient online report of selective serotonin reuptake inhibitor-induced persistent postwithdrawal anxiety and mood disorders. Psychother Psychosom 2012;81:386–388.

31 Fava GA, Gatti A, Belaise C, Guidi J, Offidani E: Withdrawal symptoms after selective serotonin reuptake inhibitors discontinuation. Psychother Psychosom 2015;84:72–81.

32 Chouinard G, Chouinard VA: New classification of selective serotonin reuptake inhibitor (SSRI) withdrawal. Psychother Psychosom 2015;84:63–71.

Chapter 18

Posttraumatic Stress Disorder

Posttraumatic stress disorder (PTSD) is a disorder that has attracted increasing attention. Its diagnostic criteria have become more complex in DSM-5 [1]. They encompass exposure to actual or threatened death, serious injury, or sexual violence; symptoms such as intrusive memories, distressing dreams, and flashbacks; persistence of avoidance of stimuli associated with the traumatic event; and alterations in cognitions, mood, arousal, and reactivity [1]. There have been various approaches under the wide umbrella of cognitive behavior therapy. They generally focus on exposure to an internal stimulus, namely the memory of the trauma [2], which can be faced by behavioral methods (imaginal exposure), cognitive restructuring, and psychoeducation, either alone or in combination (as in cognitive processing therapy), and/or associated with other techniques, such as eye movement desensitization and reprocessing and imaginal rehearsal therapy [2].

I always wondered whether making patients relive the trauma was actually necessary or if other roads to recovery could be available. I seldom see patients with PTSD in my practice. When this occurs, I do not deal with the central traumatic event, do not use imaginal exposure or debriefing, and do not generally employ psychotropic drugs. I had the chance of discussing these cases with Professor Marks, who suggested we report them in a joint publication [3]. Two patients were successfully treated with a sequential use of homework exposure fol-

Table 1. Self-observation of episodes of well-being

Situation	Well-being (0–100)	Interfering thoughts and/or behaviors	Observer
I'm walking in the city. It's a beautiful morning.	I eventually feel well. No more fears or anxiety (80).	I don't deserve this. I'm having a good time here while my colleagues must deal with difficult problems.	There are many ways to help others. The time has come for me to change my life.

lowed by Well-Being Therapy (WBT; case 1) and with WBT only (case 2). Their central trauma was discussed only in the initial history-taking session. The cases are briefly outlined here.

Case 1

Thomas was a priest aged 58 working in a mission in a developing country. One night, two burglars broke into the mission and stabbed him once. He was about to be stabbed again, probably lethally, when an outside noise made them flee. Thomas developed full-blown PTSD with vivid, repeated images day and night of the man who was going to kill him. He returned to Italy due to his PTSD and sought help there 6 months after the stabbing, as his symptoms prevented him from resuming work. He was afraid of being stabbed again whenever he went out, which severely restricted his mobility. Thomas was advised to do homework exposure to situations he avoided even in Italy (e.g., going out at night, taking a bus), which he completed. He improved greatly after 4 twice-weekly sessions, but still felt unable to resume priestly activities such as celebrating mass and taking confessions. He then began WBT. Thomas monitored and recorded periods when he felt well, thoughts which interrupted these, and cognitive restructuring of those thoughts (table 1). The patient wrote down interpretations as a potential 'observer'. After 4 sessions over 8 weeks of WBT, Thomas resumed work as a priest in a parish in Italy and showed no more general anxiety, insomnia, vivid imagery, or obvious avoidance apart from not returning to the developing world. He was repeatedly confronted with the latter, but he said he would not function as well in a mission there than in Italy. Two years after treatment, he visited his

Table 2. Self-observation of episode of well-being

Situation	Well-being (0–100)	Interfering thoughts and/or behaviors	Observer
Leaving the bank at the end of the day.	Everything went smoothly today. I was almost relaxed (70).	This was a lucky day. But luck cannot last. Anything can disclose my inadequacies.	Whenever there was an unexpected problem at work you coped with it. You've been working for 5 years now and there has been no complaint.

former mission and stayed there for 2 weeks. At the 1-year follow-up, he felt much better than before the stabbing, especially in his role of confessor. 'I learned', he said, 'that one's psychological well-being is the key: if you feel well, you transmit wellness; if you feel distressed, you transmit the gloomy view of religion which many of my colleagues have.' He remained well at his 8-year follow-up.

Case 2

Ann was a 28-year-old bank clerk who had 6 months earlier witnessed a bank robbery at her place of work. Although she had not been personally threatened, she soon developed interrupted sleep, nightmares, general anxiety, difficulty concentrating, and fear of a new robbery. As she had no avoidance, she had WBT over 8 twice-weekly sessions. She revealed in diary entries difficulties in managing everyday affairs such as dealing with nonroutine problems in her job, a fear of any unexpected event, and lack of progress and development in her work and other aspects of life. By the end of therapy, she gained a sense of mastery in dealing successfully with difficult problems at work and seeing similarities between past work difficulties and most future problems likely to arise at work (transfer of experiences). She thought it was just luck that she had not screamed or acted dangerously during the robbery. Ann was scared of any unexpected event (even a problem with a client), not just of a potential new robbery (table 2). Gaining mastery and a sense of personal growth (becoming aware that she had acquired sufficient skills to deal with unexpected problems) helped her lose her fear of a new robbery. Table 2 illustrates how she could act as an observer of her own interrupting automatic thoughts and develop alternative interpretations of them. Full remission continued at the 6-year follow-up.

Overcoming Trauma

The findings from these 2 cases should of course be interpreted with caution (the patients may have remitted spontaneously), but they are of interest because they are indicative of an alternative route to overcoming trauma and developing resilience. The role of WBT in PTSD needs to be evaluated by randomized controlled trials. However, a number of interesting observations can be made.

These cases confirm findings from a randomized controlled trial by Marks et al. [4] where exposure to central trauma memories was not found to be crucial for improvement to occur and agree with the idea that there may be varying ways to reduce fears [3]. Traumatic experiences lead people to avoid associated cues in everyday life (e.g., after a car accident they may stop driving, or avoid news on the media for fear of hearing of similar accidents). WBT's emphasis on transfer of experiences (recognition of the similarities between problems handled successfully in the past and those which are likely to come) may be instrumental in this direction [5]. Cognitive reappraisal, or the ability to cognitively reframe adverse and negative events in a positive light, is strongly associated with resilience [6]. Research on the neurobiological correlates of resilience has disclosed how different neural circuits (reward, fear conditioning and extinction, social behavior) may involve the same brain structures, in particular the amygdala, nucleus accumbens, and medial prefrontal cortex [6, 7]. Reconsolidation is a process in which old reactivated memories undergo consolidation: each time a traumatic memory is retrieved, it is integrated into an ongoing perceptual and emotional experience, which involves N-methyl-D-aspartate (NMDA) and β-adrenergic receptors, and requires cyclic adenosine monophosphate (cAMP) response-element binding protein induction [6, 7]. Singer et al. [8], on the basis of preclinical evidence, suggested that WBT may stimulate dendrite networks in the hippocampus and induce spine retraction in the basolateral amygdala (a site of storage for memories of fearful or stressful experiences), leading to a weakening of distress and traumatic memories. The pathophysiological substrates of WBT may thus be different compared to symptom-oriented cognitive behavioral strategies, reflecting that well-being and distress are not merely opposites.

WBT may thus be employed in the setting of PTSD. The 2 cases that were described used two different yet ostensibly related protocols. One is concerned with the use of behavioral intervention augmented with WBT, as described in Chapter 17 with panic and agoraphobia (the behavioral part was shorter and the total amount of sessions was 8 instead of 12). The other case involved the 8-session protocol that is described in detail in Part II of this book. It is conceivable, though yet to be tested, that WBT may also play a role in addressing adult psychological sequelae to childhood adversities [9, 10].

There has been growing awareness of the fact that traumatic experiences can also give rise to positive transformations, subsumed under the rubric of post-traumatic growth [11]. Positive changes can be observed in self-concept (e.g., new evaluation of one's strength and resilience), appreciation of new possibilities in life, social relations, hierarchy of values and priorities, and spiritual growth [12]. WBT may be uniquely suited for facilitating the process of post-traumatic growth.

References

1 Diagnostic and Statistical Manual of Mental Disorders, ed 5. Arlington, American Psychiatric Association, 2013.

2 Kulkarni M, Barrad A, Cloitre M: Post-traumatic stress disorder: assessment and treatment; in Emmelkamp PMG, Ehring T (eds): The Wiley Handbook of Anxiety Disorders, Chichester, Wiley, 2014, vol 2, pp 1078–1110.

3 Belaise C, Fava GA, Marks IM: Alternatives to debriefing and modifications to cognitive behavior therapy for post-traumatic stress disorder. Psychother Psychosom 2005;74: 212–217.

4 Marks IM, Lovell K, Noshirvani H, Livanou M, Thrasher S: Treatment of post-traumatic stress disorder by exposure and/or cognitive restructuring. Arch Gen Psychiatry 1998;55: 317–325.

5 Fava GA, Tomba E: Increasing psychological well-being and resilience by psychotherapeutic methods. J Pers 2009;77:1903–1934.

6 Southwick SM, Charney DS: The science of resilience. Science 2012;338:79–82.

7 Charney DS: Psychobiological mechanisms of resilience and vulnerability. Am J Psychiatry 2004;161:195–216.

8 Singer B, Friedman E, Seeman T, Fava GA, Ryff CD: Protective environments and health status. Neurobiol Aging 2005;265:s113–s118.

9 Faravelli C, Castellani G, Fioravanti G, Lo Sauro C, Pietrini F, Lelli L, Rotella F, Ricca V: Different childhood adversities are associated with different symptom patterns in adulthood. Psychother Psychosom 2014;83:320–321.

10 Ogrodniczuk JS, Joyce AS, Abbass AA: Childhood maltreatment and somatic complaints among adult psychiatric outpatients. Psychother Psychosom 2014;83:322–324.

11 Vazquez C, Pérez-Sales P, Ochoa C: Post-traumatic growth; in Fava GA, Ruini C (eds): Increasing Psychological Well-Being in Clinical and Educational Settings. Dordrecht, Springer, 2014, pp 57–74.

12 Tedeschi RG, Calhoun LG: The Posttraumatic Growth Inventory: measuring the positive legacy of trauma. J Trauma Stress 1996;9: 455–471.

Chapter 19
Children and Adolescents

As described in Chapter 3, a sequential treatment of fluoxetine and cognitive be-havior therapy (CBT)/Well-Being Therapy (WBT) combination was effective in reducing the risk of relapse compared to medication alone in children and adoles-cents with major depression [1]. With adolescents, the protocol described for adults in Part II can be employed. With younger age, however, substantial adapta-tions should be made. The feasibility of WBT for treating childhood psychological problems was suggested by a pilot investigation on 4 children [2]. In that trial the protocol of an 8-session child WBT was formulated [2]. Elisa Albieri and Dalila Visani [3] further elaborated that approach and expanded it to 12 sessions. Unlike what occurs with adults, psychological dimensions of well-being are introduced with a planned modality and not as the material brought by the child lends to them. I personally use a different approach that is based on my clinical experience and which provides a higher degree of flexibility, but that keeps into account insights gained from working with children [1–3]. In an early phase of my professional ca-reer I worked in a child guidance clinic [4]. Since then, I have continued to assess and treat children and adolescents, even though the bulk of my clinical practice involves adults. The WBT protocol can be suitable from the age of 8 to 14 years.

Initial Assessment

The application of the protocol should be preceded by a careful assessment. I generally see the child first alone and then I speak with either both parents (if available) or one of them. With the child, I use a circular interview that involves daily life: I review in sequence the time the child wakes up, school time, return from school, time spent home and outside, dinner, postdinner time, and quality of sleep [4]. It is circular since I return to the same times of the day and ask the same questions again. The incremental amount of information that is obtained is amazing, to the point that I may even repeat it a third time. The week review in children is repeated each time I see him/her again. My experience with children has led me to ask what patients actually do also in adult life, not limiting my assessment to symptoms that may be experienced. It is interesting how much information in terms of lifestyle [5] can be achieved by this approach. Such information supplements and refines that which can be derived by a standard interview that provides DSM criteria [6]. Treatment history, if present, is another aspect that should not be neglected.

Macroanalysis becomes particularly important with children and provides the basis for the application of WBT to this patient population. In mood and anxiety disorders, use of CBT addressing affective symptomatology generally precedes WBT, but clinical judgment should suggest the most suitable pathway. I will describe an 8-session program with 1-hour sessions once every other week, but wide variations in the number of sessions may occur. Each session may include homework assignments, games, and role-playing. The last 15 min of the session may be dedicated to the parents, when needed, particularly when behavioral suggestions are provided.

Session 1

The therapist gets the child's account of how he/she feels and current and past distress. The child is taught to identify, recognize, and express positive emotions, with the use of simple stories, animals, colors, facial expressions, and bodily gestures. The child is asked to report the positive events that happened to him/her in a diary, in a way that is similar to what occurs with adults (table 1).

Session 2

The therapist reviews the past 2 weeks and the diary, and praises the child for the work done and/or analyzes difficulties in its completion. The child is asked to remember some compliments he/she received in the past and to express his/

Table 1. Well-being diary

Situation	Well-being	Intensity[1] (0–100)
[1] 0 indicates the complete absence of well-being, while 100 indicates the most intense well-being that the child could actually experience.		

Table 2. Distress diary

Situation	Distress	Intensity[1] (0–100)
[1] 0 indicates the complete absence of distress, while 100 indicates the most intense distress that the child could actually experience.		

her feelings about them. The child is encouraged to continue the monitoring of positive life situations in the diary. It is important in this phase to take advantage of the positive reinforcement that emphasis on psychological well-being entails in children. It is crucial for the child to realize that he/she is good in certain areas and may improve his/her performance in other areas. It is also helpful to appraise whether there are optimal experiences.

Session 3

The therapist reviews the past 2 weeks and the diary, and/or analyzes difficulties in its completion. The child is asked to reflect on how it can be difficult to be nice to someone, but also how it could be gratifying to receive an unexpected compliment. The child is asked to continue the homework, adding also some negative emotions that may occur in that time frame, according to the schema provided in table 2.

Session 4

The therapist reviews the past 2 weeks and the diary, and/or analyzes difficulties in its completion. From comparing positive and negative situations, the therapist explains that the way we interpret situations can very much influence our positive or negative emotions. The child is asked to continue recording his/her positive situations in the diary only.

Session 5

The therapist reviews the past 2 weeks and the diary. The therapist looks for psychological dimensions of well-being that may apply to the material that is presented. In particular, the therapist and child try to put together a list of situations where the child displays environmental mastery, using Jahoda's broad framework [7]. The child is encouraged to add other situations in the diary and to continue recording positive situations. The changes in behavior that are requested are written in the diary as a homework assignment.

Session 6

The therapist reviews the past 2 weeks and the diary, looking for issues that may be examined according to the psychological well-being framework. In particular, the child is asked to reflect on abilities he/she already possesses and the ones he/she would like to develop. Some easy problem-solving techniques are discussed. The child is asked to continue his/her diary. The changes in behavior that are requested are written in the diary as a homework assignment.

Session 7

The therapist reviews the past 2 weeks and the diary, looking for issues that may be examined according to the psychological well-being framework. In particular, the child is asked to reflect on what type of behavior can lead to improving the way he/she feels and his/her relationship with others. The changes in behavior that are requested are written in the diary as a homework assignment.

Session 8

The therapist reviews with the child and the parents in a joint session what has been accomplished and gives practical advice on how to implement behavioral changes after the conclusion of the therapy. The child and his/her family are encouraged to call or come back whenever it is needed.

Child WBT in clinical settings at the present time has been employed in only one randomized controlled trial [1] and awaits confirmation from other adequate controlled trials. As a result, the protocol that has been outlined can be seen only as a preliminary tool.

Educational Settings

We have performed three randomized controlled trials in educational settings, which indicate that protocols based on WBT may be suitable for promoting mechanisms of resilience and psychological well-being. I owe this development to a group of coworkers (in alphabetical order: Elisa Albieri, Carlotta Belaise, Emanuela Offidani, Fedra Ottolini, Chiara Ruini, Elena Tomba, and Dalila Visani). In the first pilot study, school interventions (4 class sessions lasting a couple of hours) were performed in a population of 111 middle school students randomly assigned to: (1) a protocol using theories and techniques derived from cognitive behavioral therapy, and (2) a protocol derived from WBT. Both school-based interventions resulted in a comparable improvement in symptoms and psychological well-being [8]. This pilot investigation suggested that well-being-enhancing strategies could match CBT in the prevention of psychological distress and in promoting optimal human functioning among children.

The differential effects of the WBT and CBT approaches were subsequently explored in another controlled school intervention which involved more sessions and an adequate follow-up [9]. In this trial, 162 students attending middle schools were randomly assigned to either (1) a protocol derived from WBT or (2) an anxiety management protocol. The results of this investigation showed that WBT was found to produce significant improvements in the autonomy scale of the Psychological Well-Being Scales (PWB) [10] and in the friendliness scale of the Symptom Questionnaire (SQ) [11], whereas anxiety management ameliorated anxiety only.

WBT school interventions were extended to high school students, who are considered to be a more 'at risk' population for mood and anxiety disorders [3]. School interventions were performed in a sample of 227 students [12]. The classes were randomly assigned to either (1) a protocol derived from WBT or (2) an attention-placebo protocol, which consisted of relaxation techniques, group discussion of common problems reported by students, and conflict resolution. The WBT intervention was found to be effective in promoting psychological well-being, with particular reference to personal growth, compared to the attention-placebo protocol. Further, it was also found to be effective in decreasing distress, in particular anxiety and somatization. The beneficial effects of the WBT protocol in decreasing anxiety and somatization were maintained at the follow-up, whereas improvements faded and disappeared in the attention-placebo group [12]. The results thus indicated that WBT in educational settings may yield enduring results in terms of positive emotions and psychological well-being. The protocols that were used in these controlled studies [8, 9, 12] have been detailed elsewhere [13]. Each session is conducted by two psychologists in the presence of the teacher.

There is little doubt that WBT has great potential for children and adolescents. The main reason is the high flexibility that characterizes this age population, which lends itself to the achievement of new balances in Jahoda's terms [7]. This potential may be extended from clinical to educational settings.

References

1 Kennard BD, Emslie GJ, Mayes TL, Nakonezny PA, Jones JM, Foxwell AA, King J: Sequential treatment with fluoxetine and relapse-prevention CBT to improve outcomes in pediatric depression. Am J Psychiatry 2014;171:1083–1090.

2 Albieri E, Visani D, Offidani E, Ottolini F, Ruini C: Well-being therapy in children with emotional and behavioral disturbances: a pilot investigation. Psychother Psychosom 2009;78:387–390.

3 Albieri E, Visani D: The role of psychological well-being in childhood interventions; in Fava GA, Ruini C (eds): Increasing Psychological Well-Being in Clinical and Educational Settings. Dordrecht, Springer, 2014, pp 115–134.

4 Fava GA: Consultation psychiatry in an Italian child guidance center. Child Psychiatry Hum Dev 1981;12:90–95.

5 Tomba E: Assessment of lifestyle in relation to health; in Fava GA, Sonino N, Wise TN (eds): The Psychosomatic Assessment. Basel, Karger, 2012, pp 72–96.

6 Diagnostic and Statistical Manual of Mental Disorders, ed 5. Arlington, American Psychiatric Association, 2013.

7   Jahoda M: Current Concepts of Positive
    Mental Health. New York, Basic Books, 1958.
8   Ruini C, Belaise C, Brombin C, Caffo E, Fava
    GA: Well-being therapy in school settings: a
    pilot study. Psychother Psychosom 2006;75:
    331–336.
9   Tomba E, Belaise C, Ottolini F, Ruini C, Bra-
    vi A, Albieri E, Rafanelli C, Caffo E, Fava GA:
    Differential effects of well-being promoting
    and anxiety-management strategies in a non-
    clinical school setting. J Anxiety Disord 2010;
    24:326–333.
10 Ryff CD: Psychological well-being revisited.
    Psychother Psychosom 2014;83:10–28.
11 Kellner R: A symptom questionnaire. J Clin
    Psychiatry 1987;48:268–274.
12 Ruini C, Ottolini F, Tomba E, Belaise C, Al-
    bieri E, Visani D, Offidani E, Caffo E, Fava
    GA: School intervention for promoting psy-
    chological well-being in adolescence. J Behav
    Ther Exp Psychiatry 2009;40:522–532.
13 Visani D, Albieri E, Ruini C: School pro-
    grams for the prevention of mental health
    problems and the promotion of psychological
    well-being in children; in Fava GA, Ruini C
    (eds): Increasing Psychological Well-Being in
    Clinical and Educational Settings. Dordrecht,
    Springer, 2014, pp 177–185.

Chapter 20
New Directions

In the clinical applications that I have surveyed so far, Well-Being Therapy (WBT) was seldom used on its own. It was generally part of sequential approaches that are more in line with the complexity of psychiatric disturbances and their comorbidities. Whenever tested in a controlled fashion, WBT has been found to add incremental efficacy to the clinical approach. It is also clear that its full clinical applications are still unexplored. There are two main areas of potential development: one deals with the type of psychotherapeutic approach (whether individual, group, or family oriented) used in WBT practice, whereas the other looks into new fields of application.

Modalities of Practice

In most of the studies that have been performed, WBT has been used as a form of individual therapy. Exceptions are represented by the group therapy approach for college students performed in Iran [1] and by the school class formats in Italy [2–4]. Certainly WBT is amenable to a group format, particularly since this modality may increase sharing optimal experiences and personal meanings of psychological well-being. It is also conceivable, though yet to be tested, that WBT interventions may increase effectiveness of couple and family interventions. Kauffman and Silberman [5] have illustrated adaptations of positive psychology interventions that may improve couple therapy outcomes. Fostering the positive in relationships is indeed a target of many family and couple approaches, and elements of WBT may facilitate such a process.

At the individual level, our study on generalized anxiety disorder (GAD) [6] disclosed how, by adding monitoring of episodes of well-being, WBT may provide a more comprehensive coverage of automatic thoughts and dysfunctional schemas. As a result, WBT may be a valuable complement to any type of cognitive behavior treatment (CBT) treatment package. Such an addition may be of particular value in the high proportion of patients who fail to respond to standard pharmacological and/or psychotherapeutic treatments [7]. Compliance, both with drug treatment and psychotherapy, requires endurance and motivation [8]. It is thus conceivable that WBT may increase compliance and/or address resistances affecting progression to full recovery [9]. Indeed, clinical phenomena such as refusal to comply with basic requests are common in cognitive behavior practice.

A further issue involves the differences between WBT and other techniques that may indirectly foster psychological well-being in cognitive therapy, such as behavioral activation, schema-focused therapy, mindfulness-based cognitive therapy, acceptance and commitment therapy, and strengths-based CBT [10]. A main difference is the focus (which in WBT is on instances of emotional well-being, whereas in cognitive therapy it is on psychological distress). A second important distinction is that in cognitive therapy the goal is abatement of distress through control or contrast, whereas in WBT the goal is promotion of psychological well-being. WBT may be conceptualized as a specific strategy within the broad spectrum of self-therapies.

An additional distinction is the fact that, unlike cognitive behavioral frameworks, WBT refrains from explaining its rationale and strategies to the patient, relying instead on his/her progressive appraisal of positive self. The patient who struggles against anxiety, for instance, may be helped to view anxiety as an unavoidable element of everyday life which can be counteracted by a progressive increase in environmental mastery and self-acceptance. MacLeod and Luzon [10] wonder whether WBT can still be thought of as CBT, given its departure from the original model and different focus. The focus and the technical modalities are also quite different from positive psychology interventions [11]. Such differences also stem from the fact that WBT originated in a clinical setting to address clinical problems and its process of validation involved several randomized controlled studies. Most of the positive psychology interventions are delivered in a self-help format, sometimes in conjunction with face-to-face instructions, in very heterogeneous and nonclinical groups. Their main aim is the promotion of happiness, positive emotions, and positivity in general, which is in striking contrast with the pursuit of a balance in psychological well-being dimensions as portrayed by WBT. As illustrated in Part II of this book, an excess in positivity may be detrimental.

Further, WBT is geared to address the specific psychological dimensions of well-being that are impaired in the individual subject. As a result, there are major differences between WBT and approaches such as positive psychotherapy [12], wisdom psychotherapy [13], gratitude interventions [14], positive coaching [15], hope therapy [16], strengths-based approaches [17], forgiveness therapy [18], and quality of life therapy [19].

New Fields of Application

There are several potential areas of application of WBT that deserve to be explored, in addition to those described in the previous chapters. Some examples are described below.

Medical Disease

The need to include consideration of psychosocial factors (functioning in daily life, psychiatric and psychological symptoms, quality of life, illness behavior) has emerged as a crucial part of investigation and patient care [20]. These aspects have become particularly important in chronic diseases, where cure cannot take place, and also extend to family caregivers of chronically ill patients and health providers [20].

It is thus conceivable to postulate a role for WBT in the setting of medical disease, to counteract the limitations and challenges induced by illness experience. A randomized controlled trial, headed by Chiara Rafanelli, on addressing depressive symptoms and demoralization after myocardial infarction is currently in progress. Patients are being randomized to CBT/WBT sequential combination or clinical management. Compared to previous trials which yielded modest results in terms of prevention of cardiovascular complications [21], this investigation expands its focus to improving psychological well-being. In some way, what Chiara Rafanelli is attempting to do with patients who suffered from a myocardial infarction pertains to rehabilitation medicine, which is another important potential area of development of WBT [20]. The process of rehabilitation, in fact, requires the promotion of well-being and changes in lifestyle as primary targets of intervention [20].

Eating Disorders

Elena Tomba and her group [22] have recently documented significant impairments in psychological well-being in patients with eating disorders compared to healthy controls. This investigation, as the one that was originally performed in the residual phase of mood and anxiety disorders [23], may pave the way for assessing the value of WBT in eating disorders. WBT may particularly address body image disturbances, whether associated with eating disorders [22] or not [24, 25].

Obsessive-Compulsive Disorder

Intrusive anxiety-provoking thoughts are a core feature of obsessive-compulsive disorder [26]. Obsessive patients use punishment, worry, reappraisal, and social control as a technique of thought control more frequently than healthy subjects [27]. Punishment appears to be the strongest discriminator. Clinical observation (see Chapter 2) suggests that anxiety-provoking thoughts may often be preceded by instances of well-being in obsessive-compulsive disorder. These patients may thus have a low-threshold for well-being-related anxiety. This hypothesis needs to be tested in controlled studies and may yield innovative treatment strategies.

Psychotic Disorders

Penn and associates [28] have postulated a role for WBT in improving functional outcomes as an additional ingredient to CBT in psychotic disorders. Indeed, subjective well-being appears to be impaired in schizophrenia and is associated with reduced anterior cingulated activity during reward processing, which may induce reduced integration of environmental stimuli, motivated behavior, and reward outcome [29].

Aging

In view of the declining levels of psychological well-being with aging and the association of purpose in life with self-care [30], it is conceivable that WBT may stimulate resilience in this population. The implications of this approach, which may be pursued with both individual and group therapy interventions, are not necessarily limited to patients with medical and psychiatric comorbidities, but may be extended to the general population. The methodology of WBT group interventions that was tested in school settings may be applied also to nursing homes, residential facilities, and other places of social integration of the elderly.

References

1 Moeenizadeh M, Salagame KKK: The impact of well-being therapy on symptoms of depression. Int J Psychol Stud 2010;2:223–230.
2 Ruini C, Belaise C, Brombin C, Caffo E, Fava GA: Well-being therapy in school settings: a pilot study. Psychother Psychosom 2006;75: 331–336.
3 Tomba E, Belaise C, Ottolini F, Ruini C, Bravi A, Albieri E, Rafanelli C, Caffo E, Fava GA: Differential effects of well-being promoting and anxiety-management strategies in a non-clinical school setting. J Anxiety Disord 2010; 24:326–333.
4 Ruini C, Ottolini F, Tomba E, Belaise C, Albieri E, Visani D, Offidani E, Caffo E, Fava GA: School intervention for promoting psychological well-being in adolescence. J Behav Ther Exp Psychiatry 2009;40:522–532.
5 Kauffman C, Silberman J: Finding and fostering the positive in relationships: positive interventions in couples therapy. J Clin Psychol 2009;65:520–531.
6 Fava GA, Ruini C, Rafanelli C, Finos L, Salmaso L, Mangelli L, Sirigatti S: Well-being therapy of generalized anxiety disorder. Psychother Psychosom 2005;74:26–30.
7 Pollack MH, Otto MW, Rosenbaum JF (eds): Challenges in Clinical Practice. New York, Guilford, 1996.
8 Sirri L, Fava GA, Sonino N: The unifying concept of illness behaviour. Psychother Psychosom 2013;82:74–81.
9 Strean HS: Resolving Resistances in Psychotherapy. New York, Wiley, 1985.
10 MacLeod AK, Luzon O: The place of psychological well-being in cognitive therapy; in Fava GA, Ruini C (eds): Increasing Psychological Well-Being in Clinical and Educational Settings. Dordrecht, Springer, 2014, pp 41–55.
11 Bolier L, Haverman M, Westerhof GJ, Riper H, Smit F, Bohlmeijer E: Positive psychology interventions. BMC Public Health 2013;13: 119.
12 Seligman ME, Rashid T, Parks AC: Positive psychotherapy. Am Psychol 2006;61:774–788.
13 Linden M: Promoting resilience and well-being with wisdom and wisdom therapy; in Fava GA, Ruini C (eds): Increasing Psychological Well-Being in Clinical and Educational Settings. Dordrecht, Springer, 2014, pp 75–90.
14 Wood AM, Maltby J, Gillet R, Linley PA, Joseph S: The role of gratitude in the development of social support, stress and depression. J Res Pers 2008;42:854–871.
15 Biswas-Diener R: Personal coaching as a positive intervention. J Clin Psychol 2009;65: 544–553.
16 Geraghty AW, Wood AM, Hyland ME: Dissociating the facets of hope. J Res Pers 2010; 44:155–158.
17 Biswas-Diener R, Kashdam TB, Minhas G: A dynamic approach to psychological strength development and intervention. J Posit Psychol 2011;6:106–118.
18 Lamb S: Forgiveness therapy. J Theor Philos Psychol 2005;25:61–80.
19 Frisch MB: Quality of life therapy and assessment in health care. Clin Psychol Sci Pract 1998;5:19–40.
20 Fava GA, Sonino N: Psychosomatic medicine. Int J Clin Pract 2010;64:999–1001.
21 Rafanelli C, Sirri L, Grandi S, Fava GA: Is depression the wrong treatment target for improving outcome in coronary artery disease? Psychother Psychosom 2013;82:285–291.

22 Tomba E, Offidani E, Tecuta L, Schumann R, Ballardini D: Psychological well-being in outpatients with eating disorders. Int J Eat Disord 2014;47:252–258.

23 Rafanelli C, Park SK, Ruini C, Ottolini F, Cazzaro M, Grandi S: Rating well-being and distress. Stress Med 2000;16:55–61.

24 Phillips KA: Body dysmorphic disorder: common, severe and in need of treatment research. Psychother Psychosom 2014;83:325–329.

25 Veale D, Anson M, Miles S, Pieta M, Costa A, Ellison N: Efficacy of cognitive behaviour therapy versus anxiety management for body dysmorphic disorder. Psychother Psychosom 2014;83:341–353.

26 Marks IM: Behaviour therapy for obsessive-compulsive disorder: a decade of progress. Can J Psychiatry 1997;42:1021–1027.

27 Amir N, Cashman L, Foa EB: Strategies of thought control in obsessive-compulsive disorder. Behav Res Ther 1997;35:775–779.

28 Penn DL, Mueser KT, Tarrier N, Gloege A, Cather C, Serrano D, Otto MN: Supportive therapy for schizophrenia. Schizophr Bull 2004;30:101–112.

29 Gilleen J, Shergill SS, Kapur S: Impaired subjective well-being in schizophrenia is associated with reduced anterior cingulated activity during reward processing. Psychol Med 2015; 45:589–600.

30 Kim ES, Strecher VJ, Ryff CD: Purpose in life and use of preventive health care services. Proc Natl Acad Sci USA 2014;111:16331–16336.

Chapter 21
Going Further

The journey that I have shared with you in this book has been full of encounters with patients and colleagues, readings, and reflections. I hope that my journey may stimulate psychotherapists to embrace the perspectives entailed by Well-Being Therapy (WBT) and that these outlooks may be helpful also to physicians in general.

The first step is to pay attention to psychological well-being and to start monitoring it with patients. Those who already practice cognitive behavior therapy (CBT) should find no problem in making these first steps. WBT is mostly delivered as an additional ingredient to an array of interventions and this may facilitate its application. Its correct use, however, requires familiarity with macroanalysis, microanalysis, and the type of assessment that was detailed in Chapter 4. The full use of WBT is certainly more complex. I generally encourage colleagues who are competent psychotherapists to try it on their patients, but, as with any other psychotherapeutic technique, appropriate feedback and supervision are necessary. For these reasons I have started a process of training and certification. Information may be found at www.well-being-therapy.com.

The goal of WBT may appear ambitious. As the Latin philosopher Seneca warns in *De vita beata*, the more we look for happiness, the less likely we are to achieve it. Happiness is not everything and what is required is 'felicitatis intellectus', the awareness of well-being:

> Happy is thus the life that is in accordance to its nature, and this is possible only when the mind, first of all, is healthy at any time; then, if it is strong and energetic, definitely patient, capable of mastering everything; concerned with the body and its belongings, but without anxiety; lover of what is life, but with detachment; willing to take advantage of the gifts of fortune, without being its slave (Seneca, *De vita beata*; author's translation).

Index

Abbreviations

ACT: acceptance and commitment therapy
CBT: cognitive behavior therapy
CID: Clinical Interview for Depression
DSM: Diagnostic and Statistical Manual of Mental Disorders
GAD: generalized anxiety disorder
PTSD: posttraumatic stress disorder
PWB: Psychological Well-Being Scales
SQ: Symptom Questionnaire
SSRI: selective serotonin reuptake inhibitors
WBT: Well-Being Therapy